Action in Affirmation
Toward an Unambiguous Profession of Nursing

Project Staff for the Longitudinal Study

Jerome P. Lysaught, Ed.D.
Director

Mary Ann Christ, R.N., M.S.N.
Research Associate

Gloria A. Hagopian, R.N., Ed.D.
Research Associate

Judith Jezek, R.N., M.S.
Research Associate

Nanette L. Little, Ed.D.
Research Associate

Associates to the Staff
Diane D. Elliott, R.N., M.S.N.
Ethline I. Mais, R.N., M.S.
Laurian M. Whyte, Ph.D.

Supporting Staff
Jane DeCory, R.N.
Betty Drysdale
Jeannine Korman
Muriel Parkin

Action in Affirmation
Toward an Unambiguous Profession of Nursing

Jerome P. Lysaught, Ed.D.
Former Director
National Commission for the Study of
Nursing and Nursing Education

McGraw-Hill Book Company

New York   St. Louis   San Francisco   Auckland   Bogotá   Guatemala   Hamburg
Johannesburg   Lisbon   London   Madrid   Mexico   Montreal   New Delhi
Panama   Paris   San Juan   São Paulo   Singapore   Sydney   Tokyo   Toronto

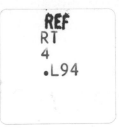

This book was set in Times Roman by Cobb/Dunlop Publisher Services, Inc.
The editor was Laura A. Dysart and
the production supervisor was Robert A. Pirrung.
R. R. Donnelley & Sons Company was printer and binder.

ACTION IN AFFIRMATION
Toward an Unambiguous Profession of Nursing

1 2 3 4 5 6 7 8 9 0   DODO   8 9 8 7 6 5 4 3 2 1 0

Library of Congress Cataloging in Publication Data

Lysaught, Jerome P
  Action in affirmation.

  Follow-up study to the original 1970 report, An abstract for action, by the National
Commission for the Study of Nursing and Nursing Education.
    1. Nursing—United States. 2. Nursing—Study and teaching—United States. 3.
National Commission for the Study of Nursing and Nursing Education. I. National
Commission for the Study of Nursing and Nursing Education. An abstract for action.
II. Title. [DNLM: 1. Education, Nursing—United States. 2. Nursing—United
States. 3. Longitudinal studies—United States. WY18 L993a]
RT4.L94   610.73'0973   80-11755
ISBN 0-07-039271-4

This investigation
was supported by the
W. K. Kellogg Foundation

It must be remembered that there is nothing more difficult to plan, more doubtful of success, nor more dangerous to manage than the creation of a new system. For the initiator has the enmity of all who would profit by the preservation of the old institution and merely lukewarm defenders in those who would gain by the new one.

Nicolo Machiavelli

O wise men, riddle me this:
    What if the dream come true?
What if the dream come true? and if
    millions unborn shall dwell
    in the house that I shaped
    in my heart.

Padraic Pearse

'Twas not for us to look for the
    fulfillment of our dream,
But it is ours to labor; ay, 'tis ours
    into our labor to translate our dreams.
Come! 'tis for those who have not sold
    their dreams
To stand together and to lead the world.

Sidney Lysaght

Contents

Foreword

One of the most important responsibilities of any grant-making organization is to regularly assess the impact of those activities to which it provides assistance. The W. K. Kellogg Foundation has learned that measuring the success of foundation-aided enterprises constitutes one of its greatest challenges. The great variety of approaches to selected issues aided by the foundation requires a matching number of evaluation techniques.

Measuring the value of a national commission is particularly difficult. To document specific changes and trends that characterize a profession is always a formidable task. The endeavor is made more complex when the concern is with modifications in both education and service and again compounded when the charge is to determine the degree to which commission recommendations influenced the changes.

Despite the formidable task it faced, the study team that produced *Action in Affirmation* has provided the foundation and those concerned with nursing education and nursing service with a meaningful analysis of the impact of the foundation-aided National Commission for the Study of Nursing and Nursing Education. The study conclusions confirm that national commissions can and sometimes do make an important contribution to the effectiveness of a profession. The study further provides clues to strengthen similar endeavors in the future and points the way to continuing developments in nursing service and education, which still fall under the heading of unfinished business. This volume should provide an important new resource for those responsible for the policies and practices that will shape the quality of nursing in the years ahead.

Robert E. Kinsinger
Vice-President
W. K. Kellogg Foundation
2 April 1980

Preface

This volume is the report of a longitudinal inquiry into the extent to which the recommendations proposed by the National Commission for the Study of Nursing and Nursing Education have been implemented over a period of 8 years. More particularly, however, it is the examination of what has happened in this regard in the 5-year period from 1973, when the Commission officially disbanded, to the end of 1978.

The report is based on information and data collected through a series of national surveys, site visits, and interviews and an examination of literature bearing on the changes that have taken place in nursing roles, education, and careers. This publication attempts to measure the progress of a number of proposals designed to make American nursing a full and effective partner in the enhancement of health care in our country. It essays this task in terms of broad movements and, in closer perspective, through the examination of 21 specific recommendations advanced by the National Commission.

Based on the findings of this investigation, there should be considerable satisfaction among those who have striven to effect change in nursing and to end the ambiguities that have plagued this profession for so long. It is hoped too that this report will encourage nurses, other health professionals, and the public who are the ultimate beneficiaries of improved nursing care to mount vigorous efforts to complete the unfinished portions of the agenda laid down by the National Commission in its first report, *An Abstract for Action.*

Over the years, many committees and commissions have attempted to study a wide variety of professions and to recommend changes in their patterns and structures that would benefit the public and increase the ability of the profession to improve its services. Frequently, these studies and reports have lain dormant and have failed to effect any significant change. The National Commission for the Study of Nursing and Nursing Education was unusual, if not unique, in its exercise of a formal 3-year implementation effort designed to initiate the process of change and to create the agencies and implements for continuing progress along prescribed dimensions. This volume, together with its predecessors, will provide theorists, researchers, and specialists in change agency with an unprecedented case history of attempted transformation involving hundreds of thousands of individuals, a multiplicity of variables, and a complex set of interrelated goals. It may well be, for these purposes, that even our failures and shortcomings can be of benefit to those who seek to engineer change in other times and other fields.

For convenience the pronoun *she* has been used throughout this book to refer nonspecifically to the nurse as a person. The author is aware that many men are also active and successful in this field and does not intend to exclude them through the traditional choice of pronoun. Neither does he mean to exclude women through the use of the terms *layman* and *manpower*, which have also been employed for the sake of convenience.

In many ways, this report has been a labor of love as well as of concern. It denotes the end of a decade of association with a remarkable group of human beings whose struggle for professionalization has profound significance for all of us who shall ever require nursing care. May this volume mark one of the last milestones on the pathway to parity for nursing in the planning, providing, and personalizing of humane health care. That situation would be the one best wish of this study staff.

To all the individuals who have been involved in the work of these 10 years, the Commissioners, the staff, and the many, many men and women who assumed responsibility for setting new directions and patterns for this, the largest of all health care professions, we trust that the record of accomplishment—though short of all our goals—is a reward in itself and contains the promise for final attainment of all that we have hoped. All your efforts have earned us that last moment of full accomplishment.

Jerome P. Lysaught
4 March 1980

Acknowledgments

For the very existence of this report and for much of the impetus toward implementation of the National Commission's recommendations, grateful acknowledgment must be made for the generous assistance of the W. K. Kellogg Foundation. Dr. Russell G. Mawby, president of the foundation, the trustees, the officers, and the staff have provided us continuing support in pursuance of the objectives outlined by the Commission, and we recognize our indebtedness to their vision and generosity.

In particular, we must mention the personal contributions of Dr. Robert Kinsinger and Barbara Lee of the foundation to our work in implementation and in evaluation. Their advice and long-suffering acceptance of academic eccentricities have helped us immeasurably in the initiation and the assessment of change processes.

We would like to thank the American Nurses' Association for its contribution of time, data, and resources to this longitudinal study. Myrtle Aydelotte, Virginia Paulson, Aleda Roth, and Naomi Patchin, as well as many others, were unstinting in their willingness to share information and materials with our staff.

Similarly, we appreciate the help of the National League for Nursing. Margaret Walsh, Margaret Sparrow, Walter Johnson, and other individuals responded helpfully to each request.

The National Joint Practice Commission, its director, William Schaffrath, and its current and former officers, Genrose Alfano, Robert Hoekelman, Otto Page, and Shirley Smoyak, were helpful in providing information throughout the course of this study.

The many institutions and individuals who participated in our surveys, site visits, interviews, and discussions are too numerous to mention individually, but we hope our gratitude is expressed in every page contained in this report.

Finally, to all the staff and to all the many people, nurses and nonnurses alike, who have fought so hard and long for the goals of the National Commission for the Study of Nursing and Nursing Education, I express my deepest appreciation. The power of dedicated human beings is both wonderful and awesome. I thank each and all of you for the privilege of experiencing these 10 years in the pursuit of a possible dream. From you I have learned faith, hope, and love in dimensions deeper than I thought existed. From you I have learned that we will overcome, and that someday there shall be an unambiguous profession of nursing playing its full role in the delivery of health care to all Americans. This final outcome cannot come soon enough.

Jerome P. Lysaught
17 March 1980

Chapter 1

Origin, Objectives, and Methods of This Investigation

In 1963, the Surgeon General's Consultant Group on Nursing issued its report entitled *Toward Quality in Nursing* [1]. The gist of this committee's recommendations was that there needed to be a national study of nursing in order to determine how best to bring that profession's needs and resources into focus. Over the next several years, the American Nurses' Foundation (ANF), the American Nurses' Association (ANA), and the National League for Nursing (NLN) sought to obtain private funding for an independent and objective inquiry into the state of the profession.

The Avalon Foundation (later renamed the Mellon Foundation), the W. K. Kellogg Foundation, and a private benefactor provided the funding for a 3-year investigation to be headed by W. Allen Wallis, then president of the University of Rochester. In 1970, the report of the National Commission for the Study of Nursing and Nursing Education (NCSNNE) was published as *An Abstract for Action* [2]. In this volume, the Commission and staff reported their findings and recommendations for the repatterning of nursing roles, education, and career perspectives. Through related developments in all three of these strands, the National Commission sought to make American nursing a full and unambiguous profession capable of serving as a principal partner in the enhanced delivery of health care to our people.

Even before the appearance of a supplementary volume, *An Abstract for Action:*

1

Appendices [3], in 1971, the Commission had made a basic decision concerning the future of its recommendations. Reviewing the several previous studies of nursing in the United States, which at that point stretched back almost 50 years, the Commissioners resolved to see that there would be a formal implementation effort mounted to ensure that the proposals were at least heard and debated and that a beginning could be made on the many tasks proposed for reorganizing this, the largest of our health practitioner professions.

Accordingly, the W. K. Kellogg Foundation, the American Nurses' Association, and the National League for Nursing funded a 3-year continuation of the National Commission for the express purpose of laying a foundation for broad-scale change. The Commission itself was enlarged. Those original members who felt they had to leave the group were asked to participate in an advisory council that would aid in the implementation effort but would make a limited time demand upon members. The president of the Commission for the second phase of activities was Leroy E. Burney, M.D., then president of the Milbank Memorial Fund.*

From 1970 through 1973, the Commission, its staff, and a host of advisory groups, regional associates, and volunteers set out to inform nurses, physicians, administrators, public agencies, private groups, and the lay public about the strengths and the flaws that had been discovered in nursing and the rationale behind the changes that were proposed to strengthen the profession's contribution to our health care system. A full report on the activities, the successes, and the disappointments of that period was published in *From Abstract into Action* in 1973 [4], and a complementary volume, *Action in Nursing* [5], provided an anthology of monographs and articles prepared by the Commission staff as well as papers relating to the Commission's recommendations written by independent critics and advocates of our positions.

These third and fourth volumes in the series of Commission writings marked the formal close of the 6-year study and implementation period as well as the legal termination of the Commission itself. In anticipation of this closing, the staff was requested to draw up a plan for a longitudinal study of the impact of the National Commission for the Study of Nursing and Nursing Education on health care through an examination of the extent of implementation of its recommendations over time. Accordingly, the staff drew up a set of speculative statements concerning the anticipated results on 21 key recommendations in which there could be shown both concomitant variation and a temporal relationship—such that one could say with some certainty either that this action began with a specific Commission proposal or that the Commission's activities as recorded in the materials on the implementation period had specific influence on reported outcomes.

In all, the original Commission had proposed more than 60 recommendations for the improvement of American nursing. By limiting the longitudinal study to a subset of 21, the staff sought to eliminate any of these proposals that might well have been subject to general events of the times or to movements set into motion even as the investigation was under way.

---

*The membership of the Commission and the advisory council is presented in the frontmatter of the volume *From Abstract into Action,* McGraw-Hill Book Company, New York, 1973.

The intention of the longitudinal study, in the minds of Commission members and staff, was never to serve as a self-congratulatory instrument in the event of success or as a disclaimer or excusatory document in the event of disappointment. Rather, the study was to function as nearly as possible as an objective statement of outcomes in such a way that any other committee or commission seeking to study a profession and effect change and innovation might take all our reports in sequence; trace each effort, each strategy, and each alternative choice; and compare these with the overall results achieved. Out of this explication and documentation, it was hoped, might come greater knowledge than any of us had as we embarked on the successive stages of study, implementation, and follow-up. For those recommendations for which implementation was highly successful, our strategy may be examined with confidence. Where there was failure, let others profit by our errors of commission and omission. That is our purpose in this work.

This volume, then, is intended for *students of nursing,* including nursing students, practitioners, faculty members, researchers, and all others. It is intended to help physicians, administrators, health planners, and others who need to know more about this large group of care providers. This volume, though, in companionship with its predecessors, is also intended for students of social and organizational change of any discipline who seek to examine professional phenomena. We have hoped to portray as accurately and clearly as possible the information on which recommendations were based, the intended outcome of each proposal, the activities aimed at marshaling support, and, over time, the measurement of actual results.

From the outset of our involvement, the Commission and the staff knew that some proposals for professional reorganization, like those of Flexner in the field of medicine, had been successfully enacted. Most other professional studies, like the previous inquiries into nursing, had been successful in quite limited ways if at all. We tried to develop both strategic and tactical plans from what we perceived were the high-probability change models and avoided low-probability precedents. If other planners and change agents could benefit from our experience, then the National Commission would have proved valuable in a significant dimension.

Let it be added, however, that the objective reporting of success and failure does not detract from our original concerns for the repatterning of American nursing. Every one of the many recommendations of the original Commission was part of a conceptual framework that envisaged a new, fully professional House of Nursing with expanded roles in client care across the whole broad range of client need. Nursing education was to be strengthened, made into a system, and reunited with practice so that students would interact with faculty models of clinical excellence. Nursing careers were to be made rewarding and self-actualizing so that practitioners might find in their lifework a constant renewal of that intrinsic drive that brought them into the profession initially. So, this study staff finds exhilaration in the areas of success, and we are disappointed in the areas of limited implementation and failure.

Further, we would still urge nursing—its individuals and its organizations—to examine the record of accomplishments and shortcomings and resolve that from this record should be constructed its agenda for the eighties. Full professionalization, full partnerhood in health care delivery, and full realization of the conceptual framework of the National Commission are goals surely worth achieving. This volume will attempt to specify wherein we have reached or failed each mark, and from that point nursing can, if it chooses, press on to the full attainment of each element still unmet.

INITIATION OF THIS INVESTIGATION

In 1976, the plan for the longitudinal follow-up of the National Commissions's recommendations was submitted to the W. K. Kellogg Foundation together with a proposal for funding for a 1-year period. The evaluation would be conducted out of the University of Rochester using doctoral students and graduate assistants of that institution to aid in carrying out the inquiry protocols. Upon approval, the follow-up study actually was begun in December of 1977 with an anticipated completion target of 1978. For a variety of reasons, including the need to work largely during academic semesters, when graduate assistants were available, and the natural delays in effecting the transmission and return of surveys and questionnaires, the grant from the Kellogg Foundation for the evaluation was modified to permit completion of the project and report in 1979. This extension had the added virtue of permitting the study staff to assess a full 5-year period of data and information, from 1973 through 1978. From the standpoint of the longitudinal protocols, the study's extension simply meant an editorial revision of the statements of expectation. For the purposes of measurement, it allowed us some increased assurance that maturation in implementation had taken place and that peaks or valleys of activity in the first few months after the Commission had closed its offices had been smoothed out over a longer intervening period.

METHODOLOGY OF THE INVESTIGATION

The plans for the longitudinal evaluation of activity called for a normative, descriptive examination of the extent of implementation recorded in 21 specific areas together with a more general appraisal of the scope of change in the 3 divisions of the initial inquiry: nursing roles and functions, nursing education, and nursing careers.

Over the period from December 1977 through May 1978, the director of the study, working with doctoral assistants and with the help of other interested graduate students, conducted a general bibliographic search of materials published between 1973 and 1979, with an emphasis on articles and research reports related to the 21 propositions for change. This research was supplemented by a series of visits to and interviews in health care facilities, educational institutions, and statewide implementation activities. The major source of information on the extent of movement, however, was derived from a series of surveys and questionnaires presented to nursing organizations and facilities. These surveys and questionnaires included:

  1   A survey of all state nurses' associations which inquired into such areas as the activity of state master planning committees and joint practice groups

2   A survey of a stratified sample of 264 educational institutes for nursing education, including all varieties of preparatory programs

3   A survey of 185 hospitals and in-patient care facilities to determine the current configurations of clinical care and the introduction of such positions as clinical specialists and certified practitioners

4   A survey of nursing students conducted in collaboration with the National Students' Nursing Association, from which 600 random returns were drawn in accordance with current admission figures, to provide a striated sample

5   A survey of nurse specialty practice organizations to determine their activities in fields such as certification, continuing education, and professional issues

To flesh out the information developed from these surveys, visits were made to the American Nurses' Association, the National League for Nursing, the federal Division of Nursing, the National Joint Practice Commission (NJPC), the American Hospital Association, and a number of other associations, including some of the nurse specialty practice groups. Over the duration of the evaluation study, staff personnel from ANA, NLN, and the Division of Nursing frequently provided additional information and material and assisted our graduate assistants in the collection of bibliographic information and data.

Over the period from May through September 1979, the director of the study utilized the draft statements and analyses that had been developed in collaboration with the staff and began the process of developing the manuscript for the final report. The report was updated as closely as possible through the summer of 1979 and even within the month of September as developments occurred that might relate to the general environment of professional nursing. The data on the specific recommendations and their implementation, however, were based entirely on information and statistics through December 1978.

MEMBERSHIP OF THE STUDY STAFF

Over the period of the evaluation study, four doctoral assistants worked on specific projects and inquiries related to the longitudinal investigation. In addition, other graduate students, not all of them nurses, used elements of our work to derive materials for qualifying papers and dissertations. The contributions of our appointees and our volunteers lay in these areas:

Nanette L. Little, Ed.D., conducted much of the preliminary work in bibliographic collection and in the planning of site visits and interviews. Her doctoral dissertation on the "Characteristics and Role Perceptions of Graduates of Baccalaureate Dental Hygiene Programs in the United States" [6] was designed to replicate some of the original NCSNNE instruments and hypotheses with another professional group that shares a number of related problems and concerns in common with nursing.

Gloria A. Hagopian, R.N., Ed.D., performed the analysis of the questionnaires of the state nurses' associations as well as a companion analysis of those nine states that had comprised the original pilot or target group for purposes of the formal implementation period. Her doctoral dissertation on "The Nursing Deanship: Administrative Problems and Educational Needs" [7] was initiated in part by her interest in the materials on education and leadership that she reviewed for the evaluation study.

Mary Ann Christ, R.N., M.S., analyzed the returns from the educational institutions and, with help from Dr. Hagopian, completed the analysis of surveys from the directors of nursing service. Her dissertation on "Research Priorities in a Nursing Unification Model" [8], which is currently nearing completion, is an effort to examine certain implications of the recombination of nursing education with practice in centers utilizing this organizational concept.

Judith Jezek, R.N., M.S., was also assigned specifically to the evaluation project and essentially committed her assistantship activities for two semesters to the furtherance of our analyses and draft positions. In particular, she authored two papers on "The Funding of Nursing Research" [9] and "Financing of Nursing Education: Past and Future" [10], which were instrumental in our assessment of those areas for inclusion in this evaluational report. A matriculated doctoral student, she plans to use the work with the study staff in the development of her doctoral dissertation.

Laurian M. Whyte, Ph.D., was not connected directly with the evaluation study, but became interested in the emerging programs for certification of advanced nursing practice. Her interaction with other graduate students was of great value, and her dissertation on "The Effect of Certification on the Wages and Hours Worked by Critical Care Nurses" [11] is the first systematic assessment of the economics of certification.

Ethline Mais, R.N., is a graduate student in the adult learning program of the university. In a study of professionalism and professionalization, she undertook a review of early professionalization in American nursing and, in particular, prepared an analysis of the differences between the Nightingale proposal for model systems of nursing education and practice and the American adaptation of those plans [12].

The combined efforts and writings of these individuals not only contributed to the longitudinal follow-up of the National Commission's implementation efforts, but also initiated the development of new knowledge in areas of great importance to the continuing professionalization of nursing. In particular, the doctoral dissertations, those completed and those nearing completion, deserve examination by the profession for their insights into role execution, educational patterning, and career perspectives.

USE OF CRITICAL READERS

As a way of checking the interpretation and analyses of the director and the study staff, arrangements were made to utilize a number of experienced nurse leaders as critical readers and commentators. These individuals were furnished with draft chapters of the final report in particular areas of specialty, and their comments, criticisms, and suggestions were invited. Each draft chapter was then reviewed in the light of the responses, and appropriate adjustments were made or additional data provided to clarify or explicate each point suggested by a reviewer. Our readers included:

Myrtle K. Aydellotte, Ph.D., executive director, American Nurses' Association
Rose Marie Chioni, Ph.D., dean, University of Virginia School of Nursing
Rheba de Tornyay, Ed.D., dean, University of Washington School of Nursing
Carol A. Lindeman, Ph.D., dean, University of Oregon School of Nursing
Martha Mitchell, M.S.N., director, Connecticut Mental Health Center

The comments and suggestions proffered by the readers were particularly helpful in enabling us to sharpen points and consider alternative interpretations of data analysis. Their contributions materially aided in the final draft of this report, and the staff expresses its appreciation for their help. The final responsibility, however, for the publication rests with the director, and his is the burden of commission or omission.

INVOLVEMENT OF FORMER COMMISSIONERS

At the beginning of the study period, the former commissioners from both the investigative and implementation phases were informed of the undertaking and received a copy of the plan that had been drawn up in 1973.* As the results and draft position papers were being drawn together in the spring of 1979, a series of three small group meetings were planned for Chicago, Atlanta, and Los Angeles so that the former Commissioners might be able to discuss the findings and review the report in a preliminary fashion. Despite their busy schedules and other commitments—not to mention the fact that their obligations had truly expired several years ago—7 of the 19 Commissioners were able to make one of the meetings, and others made arrangements to speak individually with the director and chat informally about the progress that had been recorded.

Although it was impossible to have all the Commissioners meet together—or even to include all of them in the small group sessions—we have enjoyed their interest and support and the confident knowledge that when we called on any one of them for information or assistance, it was provided immediately. The Commissioners bear no responsibility for this report, but they deserve recognition for the many contributions they have made to the implementation effort and to the attainment of many of the objectives marked out for accomplishment.

AN OUTLINE OF THIS REPORT

In the succeeding chapters, we will present a series of observations, data, and analyses that are deliberately constructed so as to parallel the original commentaries and proposals in *An Abstract for Action.* Chapter 2 deals with the status of nursing on the American health care scene and attempts to assess the differences that can be seen from the picture of 1968. Chapter 3 is an analysis of the characteristics and scope of nursing practice along with an exposition of the conceptual framework

*For information on the national commissioners during both the investigative and the implementation stages, see Chapter 1 in *An Abstract for Action* [1] and Chapter 1 in *From Abstract into Action* [3].

advanced by the National Commission in 1970 and an updated consideration of its implications. Chapter 4 is a discussion of our findings relative to the implementation of recommendations for nursing roles and practice. Chapter 5 treats the implementation of recommendations for nursing education. Chapter 6 deals with the implementation of recommendations for the enhancement of nursing careers. Chapter 7 is a presentation and summary analysis of the 21 specific recommendations that were selected by the study staff in 1973 and approved by the National Commission for the Study of Nursing and Nursing Education as the basis for this longitudinal study.

For readers' convenience, the same general division of materials and concepts is utilized in the formats of *From Abstract into Action* and *Action in Nursing* so that a parallelism is built into each stage of the Commission's work. This structuring should not only assist nurses in their use of these publications but also make them more useful to other researchers whose fields of interest might be limited to one or two of the areas touched on in the broad considerations of the National Commission.

Readers should note that the conditions described in this book are those that existed in 1979 at the completion of the project.

REFERENCES

1   "Toward Quality in Nursing," *Report of the Surgeon General's Consultant Group on Nursing,* U.S. Department of Health, Education, and Welfare, PHS Publication 992, Washington, D.C., 1963.

2   Jerome P. Lysaught, *An Abstract for Action,* McGraw-Hill Book Company, New York, 1970.

3   Jerome P. Lysaught, *An Abstract for Action: Appendices,* McGraw-Hill Book Company, New York, 1971.

4   Jerome P. Lysaught, *From Abstract into Action,* McGraw-Hill Book Company, New York, 1973.

5   Jerome P. Lysaught (ed.), *Action in Nursing: Progress in Professional Purpose,* McGraw-Hill Book Company, New York, 1974.

6   Nanette L. Little, "Characteristics and Role Perceptions of Baccalaureate Dental Hygiene Programs in the United States," unpublished doctoral dissertation, The University of Rochester, Rochester, N.Y., 1977.

7   Gloria A. Hagopian, "The Nursing Deanship: Administrative Problems and Educational Needs," unpublished doctoral dissertation, The University of Rochester, Rochester, N.Y., 1979.

8   Mary Ann Christ, "Research Priorities in a Nursing Unification Model," proposal for a doctoral dissertation, Center for Educational Administration, Graduate School of Education and Human Development, The University of Rochester, Rochester, N.Y., 1978.

9   Judith Jezek, "The Funding of Research," unpublished position paper, Center for Educational Administration, Graduate School of Education and Human Development, The University of Rochester, Rochester, N.Y., 1979.

10 Judith Jezek, "Financing of Nursing Education: Past and Future," unpublished qualifying paper, Center for Educational Administration, Graduate School of Education and Human Development, The University of Rochester, Rochester, N.Y., 1979.

11 Laurian M. Whyte, "The Effect of Certification on the Wages and Hours Worked by Critical Care Nurses," unpublished doctoral dissertation, The University of Rochester, Rochester, N.Y., 1979.
12 Ethline Mais, "Nursing Professionalization in America," unpublished position paper, Center for Educational Administration, Graduate School of Education and Human Development, The University of Rochester, Rochester, N.Y., 1979.

Chapter 2

Nursing on the American Health Scene

In 1970, the National Commission for the Study of Nursing and Nursing Education (NCSNNE) presented, in *An Abstract for Action,* a brief review of the historical development of nursing and nursing education in the United States. From the establishment of the Nightingale School of Nursing in London in 1860, there was interest in the development of training programs for skilled attendants to assist physicians in the care of patients. It was, in fact, a committee of the American Medical Association (AMA) that first proposed that district schools be established across the country to supply sufficient numbers of nurses to accommodate the needs of hospitals. In 1872, the first finishing class of "trained nurses" graduated from the New England Hospital for Women and Children. In the following year, so-called Nightingale schools were established at Bellevue, New Haven, and Massachusetts General hospitals.

There were some obvious benefits to society and to the graduates of these programs, but there were problems as well. The development of the early nursing programs, limited as most were to female applicants helped to engrave in stone the sexual stereotyping of medicine and nursing in this country. Early female graduates of medical colleges often found themselves forced to function as nurses because of resistance to their obtaining licensure and hospital privileges. The systematic exclusion of men from nursing was not offset to any great extent by the opening of a few nurse training programs for males only. Today, we graduate about 5 men for every 100 women from our preparatory institutions for nursing. Of our nurses in practice, the percentage of males is about half the figure represented by male graduates— approximately 3 percent.

There were, however, even more profound shortcomings in the American adaptation of the Nightingale plan for nursing education and practice than the restraint on admitting males into the schools. Table 2-1 provides a comparison of the model proposed by the English proponent of professional nursing and the actuality of our implementation [1]. Nightingale's plan was never implemented to her complete satisfaction in England, and although some of the American hospital schools evolved in ways that are approximations to her ideals, the general level of adaptation was poor.

Between 1872 and 1932, the number of hospital training programs grew from 1 to 1844. There was no way to provide quality in faculty or selectivity in students. It was not until 1899 that the first series of courses for graduate nurses was established, at Teachers College, Columbia University, to provide some professional background in teaching for nurse faculty members.

The control of the hospital, both financial and administrative, over the school ensured both the ascendance of the medical service model as the curricular standard for the nurse training school and the organizational subordination of the nurse to

Table 2-1 Comparison of Proposed and Characteristic Adaptations of the Nightingale Plan for Professional Nursing

Nightingale model	American adaptation
Nursing education	
1. Nursing educators and students carefully selected	1. Scarcity of qualified educators; little selectivity in students
2. Nursing taught and controlled by nurses	2. Nurses nominally in charge of program but obligated to hospital
3. Nursing schools to be autonomous and financially independent	3. Nursing schools neither autonomous nor financially independent
4. Careful contractual arrangements with clinical facilities for the purpose of practical training	4. Hospitals required student nurse service in exchange for experience and based on institutional needs
5. Research-oriented teaching faculty to explore nursing practice	5. Little or no research orientation: emphasis on pragmatic skills
6. Provision for continuing education and upgrading of practice	6. Little or no provision for education beyond preparation
Nursing practice	
1. Holistic approach to role	1. Task-oriented approach to role
2. Client-centered orientation	2. Institution-centered orientation
3. Two-component system of care: a. Health nursing—preventive care b. Sick nursing—care of the ill	3. One-component system of care: a. Sick nursing—care of the ill b. Approach based on medical-service model
4. Nursing process emphasized as a scientific approach	4. Nursing process emphasized as a reactive process in response to physician order and institutional regulations

the physician and the administrator. So deeply embedded is this concept of relationships that, in late 1978, a proposal by the National Joint Practice Commission (NJPC)
to have organized professional nursing staffs of hospitals be directly accountable to
the governing board of the hospital was considered most objectionable by committees and councils of the American Hospital Association (AHA) [2]. No one questions the right of medical service to have access to the governing board; few would
presume that the administrator has greater knowledge about medicine than a physician. Yet, hospital administrators historically have held power and authority over
nursing.

Not only in the educational aspects of the Nightingale plan did the American
adaptation suffer. Much of the holistic approach to client care and, in particular, the
concept of a two-component system of care that provided nursing support to the well
and to the sick was largely discarded in favor of a task-oriented, illness-centered
approach. In short, the Nightingale plan envisaged the nurse as a professional
collaborator; the American approach developed an aide for the physician and an
employee for the administrator. The implications have been far-reaching.

In its analysis of American nursing, the National Commission examined the
slow process by which it evolved from essentially a vocation, through an occupation,
and into the status of a near, or minor, profession. Throughout the more than 100
years of formal preparation and socialization into the practice of nursing, the early
patterns of subordination and task orientation have continued to shape and to
influence both education and practice. Over generations that were quite comfortable
with a concept of male authority and female weakness, this concept had all the
ingredients of a self-fulfilling prophecy. Nor, it must be added, were many nurses
upset by the roles in which they were cast. Many saw nursing as a fine preparation
for marriage and family life; few tended to view it as a lifelong career. Many nurses
were content to let physicians and administrators carry the responsibility and the
liability for decision making and were satisfied in caring for a patient essentially in
terms of the orders and the charts.

The point has been made that medicine and nursing were, in important ways,
more alike in 1900 than many physicians—or the public—might think. At that time,
only 5 medical colleges out of more than 160 institutions required a college degree.
Most of the schools for physician training were proprietary institutions that emphasized didactic teaching. The body of knowledge to guide practice was severely
limited, and only about 20 percent of the cases presenting to a physician were treated
with a scientific regimen of care. Nevertheless the physician was socialized to be
superordinate to the nurse and to be independent in decision making. With the
published report of the Flexner [3] study in 1910, however, the relationship of
medicine and nursing became essentially different.

As a result of Flexner's recommendations, medical education became firmly
embedded in the university structure for higher education. Rigorous training in the
biological sciences became a requirement, and clinical instruction took place in the
wards and the clinics as well as in the lecture hall. Admission standards were raised,
state board (and, later, national board) examinations became more challenging, and
the number of medical schools was reduced largely through the demise of the

proprietary institutions. The result was a remarkable upgrading in physician quality, the elaboration of a germ theory that strengthened the armamentarium of the practitioner in both the cure and the prevention of illness, and the encouragement of research into deeper dimensions of knowledge and understanding. Within 70 years we have transformed the entire scope and measure of American medicine and of the physicians who practice within its domain.

This growth was accompanied by another phenomenon as well. In opting for a scientific and disciplined educational base for medicine, Flexner and his followers argued essentially for the development of an elite—a body of physicians whose superior knowledge and dedication rightfully entitled them to autonomy, self-regulation, and widened authority over the governance of their profession. With this companion development, Flexner hoped to attract the brightest and most dedicated individuals possible to the challenge of medical training and practice, through a combination of social reward and personal fulfillment. In this effort he was eminently successful, although critics have pointed out that socioeconomic determinism also played a major role in the process through restricting poorer individuals from applying to the longer and much more expensive preparatory programs and encouraging others to see medicine as an inviting capital investment with great promise of financial reward at the end of the training period.

Between 1910 and 1923, the differences in the relationship between medicine and nursing became pronounced. Even as the knowledge base of medicine widened the gap between the two, so the early emergence of the new elite had a profound impact on the dynamics of daily relationships. This increasing distance provided part of the impetus for the first national study of nursing, the Goldmark Commission, which inquired into the practice and education of nursing and advocated improvements that would have moved the body along a path parallel to that taken by medicine. The development of collegiate education for nurses, the emphasis on an enlarged knowledge base to guide practice, and the proposal of nonhospital components in nursing care all would have helped to readjust the balance of nursing with medicine and at a point well above the locus for both groups in 1900. Most of the proposals of the Goldmark study [4]—in contrast to those of Flexner—went quietly to rest in a sea of benign indifference. The more than 1700 hospital schools of nursing were content to conduct business as usual, and few physicians or administrators had any vision of the contribution that a fully professional nurse might make to the improvement of care. In short, the American adaptation of the Nightingale plan won out—almost without a contest.

In retrospect, as one considers a conceptual schema for the analysis of professional values and motives, it is possible to plot the growing separation that took place between medicine and nursing after 1900. In Figure 2–1, we can conceive of two axes that relate to important dimensions of professionalization. On the vertical axis we can contrast the difference in knowledge base between what is essentially an idiosyncratic system of beliefs and guesses and one based on the systematic collection of data, experimentation, and rigorous analysis. After 1900, the thrust of American medicine was deliberately guided—even forced—from folk practice to rigorous inquiry. Nursing continued to emphasize task learning and the art of caring. On the

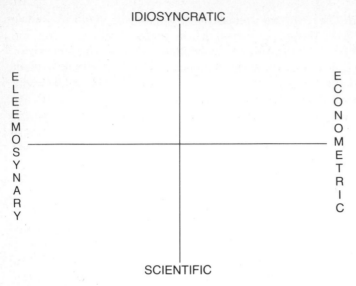

Figure 2-1   Conceptual schema for analysis of professional values and motives.

horizontal axis we see medicine, even though Flexner for one predicted a great increase in altruism, becoming more caught up in the economics of professional development. Costs of education are increasing; so, too, must the return on the investment. As largely independent practitioners, physicians are free to set fees and to demand that hospitals provide them with the equipment, the laboratories, and the assisting personnel that will permit the acceleration of both knowledge and clinical application. Nurses, meanwhile, still operate on the eleemosynary concept that there is an essentially unlimited need for their services which is unrelated to any intersection of supply and demand curves. While the number of medical schools decreased significantly in the first three decades after the Flexner report, the number of preparatory programs in nursing continued to rise until the adverse effects of the depression years caused the demise of the financially marginal institutions. Later, with the advent of associate degree programs in community colleges, we again saw a spectacular growth rate with, only recently, a plateauing at the level of 1375 preparatory programs. In 1900, there were approximately 3 schools of nursing for each medical college; in 1978, there were more than 12.

Over much of this period of time, up to the Second World War, and in periods after, we experienced a physician shortage and a nursing surplus. Income for physicians was increased as demand exceeded supply. Salaries for nurses were depressed when supply exceeded demand. Moreover, the dependent status of the nurse in relation to the hospital and the ability of regional groups of hospitals to function as oligopolies meant that a free market did not exist and that, when local nursing shortages occurred, the salary level most often remained fixed and other expedients, such as the recruitment of aides, attendants, and orderlies, were substituted for the registered nurse. It must be added, however, that directors of nursing service not only acquiesced in these matters, for the most part, but also busied themselves in the training of substitutes and lesser-skilled personnel as part of their "human-itarian" duty.

Today, we still find, in the face of conflicting information about a shortage of nurses, an atmosphere that constantly emphasizes the supply component of the manpower equation and has almost no concern for the rates of retention and with-drawal or for the reality of the demand that actually exists within the health care system. The net effect is that nursing has seldom moved with vigor toward the econometric end of the horizontal scale that might emphasize the need for adequate reward structures and the development of a true career perspective in which practi-tioners might look toward a satisfying lifetime of involvement.

One inevitable result of the experiences of medicine and nursing since 1910 is that, in terms of the schema presented in Figure 2–1, physicians have moved emphat-ically into the lower right quadrant, with a heavy emphasis on research and science coupled with a heightened recognition of the economic considerations involved in care and compensation. Some would say that the current plot point represents too heavy a concern with the malady and too little concern with the client as a human being; others would add that the economics of medicine and health care have become unreasonably in favor of the provider and practitioner at the expense of the patient. Nevertheless, there is evidence, too, of the altruism that Flexner had hoped would follow from his development of a meritocracy.

Over this same course of years, nursing has largely confined itself to the upper left quadrant, maintaining its many preparatory programs and recruiting students even when some economists have argued that the net effect of these activities is to depress nursing salaries below that of other groups with far less training or responsi-bility of performance. Relatedly, the knowledge base of nursing has shown only small incremental gains. The content of many preparatory programs in nursing education is not appreciably different from the curriculum of 10 years ago and perhaps before that. The change that has occurred is more often due to the impact of increased technology than the reformulation of nursing roles based on experimen-tal inquiry and an expanded corpus of data. Certainly, there are and have been many nurses at the cutting edge of role enlargement and there have been those who urged reconsideration of reward systems and career patterns, but the strong voices calling for professionalization are demonstrably in the minority and face as much opposition and rancor, at times, from their colleagues as ever they receive from physicians and health administrators.

In attempting to describe and to deal with this general malaise, the National Commission recommended a series of changes in nursing education and practice that do, indeed, bear a resemblance to the idealized Nightingale model as well as to the full professions of our society. In examining the recent historical development of medicine, the commissioners hoped to bridge the gulf between our two largest clinical practitioner groups by encouraging change on both their parts, but neces-sarily through greater movement on the part of nursing. By building closer relation-ships between nurses and physicians, by making nursing more scientific and career-oriented without losing the humaneness and altruism that should character-ize a consulting profession, we hoped to build a whole new framework for the delivery of health care effectively, efficiently, and with deep concern for the client and consumer. To do this, however, requires an examination of the general standards by which any full profession can be measured.

CHARACTERISTICS OF AMERICAN NURSING TODAY

In the literature on professions and professionalism, many criteria have been advanced for the analysis of an occupation to determine its qualifications for being called a *profession.* In Figure 2–2, you will see six statements that are almost universally applied to the consideration of professionalism; the first five of those were reviewed systematically in *An Abstract for Action,* and the sixth was treated in the concluding chapter of that report almost in the form of a summary and call to action. In the following sections of this chapter, we will reconsider these characteristics in light of the years intervening between 1970 and 1978 and for the purpose of developing a general understanding of the present status of nursing as a full profession. More detailed examination of the specifics of change in education, practice, and careers will be taken up in succeeding chapters of this report.

Strong Level of Commitment

When the National Commission began its investigation into American nursing, there were over 1,100,000 persons who had achieved licensure as registered nurses. Of these, some 909,000 maintained their licenses, but over 30 percent were unemployed in nursing and, of those who were working, almost 25 percent were part-time, so that our full-time nurses represented 445,300 persons, or approximately 40 percent of the total "supply." Over the period from 1973 to 1978, no less than 376,955 graduations were reported from basic registered nurse training programs. Yet in 1978, our best approximations indicated that there was little change in the distribution patterns between the employed and the unemployed, with a slight shift toward part-time practice within the employed group. If we project on straight-line increments our experience since 1966, we would expect to find a configuration of nursing employment in 1980 generally divided according to the areas portrayed in Figure

1. Strong Level of Commitment

2. Long and Disciplined
   Educational Process

3. Unique Body of Knowledge and Skill

4. Discretionary Authority and Judgment

5. Active and Cohesive
   Professional Organization

6. Acknowledged Social Worth   **Figure 2–2**   General characteristics of
   and Contribution   American professions.

2–3. Fifty percent of the total supply of American nursing will be uninvolved in nursing practice: this group will be almost equally divided between those who do not maintain a license and those who maintain one but do not use it. The employed nurses will be split on roughly a one-third to two-thirds ratio, with the greater number being employed fulltime. (It should be noted that the figures used by this study staff and the Manpower Department of the American Nurses' Association differ in one significant point. The ANA, rightfully for its purpose, generally concerns itself with only those nurses who maintain a license. For our purposes, it is essential to recognize that historical and actuarial data indicate that fully one out of every four American registered nurses divests herself of licensed status before the point of normal retirement or anticipated inactivity. This situation, of course, has profound implications for supply and for the level of professional commitment.)

A recent survey conducted by United Press International (UPI) sought to spotlight reasons for the withdrawal of nurses from the practice of their profession [5]. The general pattern derived is consistent with the findings of this study staff and with several other contemporary analyses of nursing on the American health scene. Among the feelings that UPI reported were these: inadequate financial compensation both in relation to other occupations and in terms of incremental increases based on greater experience and enlarged competency; the limitations placed on the role performance and expanded practice of nurses by traditional job standards and physician expectations; the stress of dealing with the complexities of care in our present era of increased technology and intricate praxis; and the emotional burnout experienced by many individuals who find it draining to cope with the critically and terminally ill in many major hospitals and medical centers day in and day out.

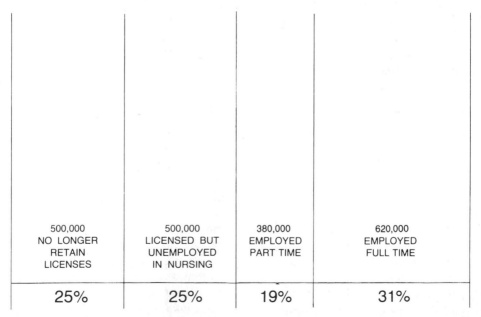

500,000 NO LONGER RETAIN LICENSES	500,000 LICENSED BUT UNEMPLOYED IN NURSING	380,000 EMPLOYED PART TIME	620,000 EMPLOYED FULL TIME
25%	25%	19%	31%

Figure 2–3 Estimates on employment status of nurses, 1980.

Comparative figures on turnover rates for nursing indicate that they still are far higher than those of teachers, other health professionals, or licensed practical nurses. Undoubtedly this phenomenon is related to the reasons cited for withdrawal; turnover seemingly represents a search for more satisfying alternatives that, unfortunately, may not exist.

Actually the turmoil within the ranks of nursing has been masked by the fact that, between 1970 and 1976, the graduations from basic nursing programs increased by nearly 80 percent. From 1976 through 1978, that figure essentially leveled off, as did the figure for admittances. This leveling off means that over the next several years we must address the matter of commitment and retention more seriously than ever before.

If we are to develop a nursing resource sufficient to meet our requirements within the health care delivery system, we must construct a reward system that is not only competitive but also career-oriented, that is, scaled to reward increased clinical competency and leadership in practice. We must further give room to the expansion of scope in nursing roles to encourage the bright and the motivated to find satisfaction in a growing contribution to care rather than experiencing frustration from the imposition of an unanalyzed ceiling on their behavior. In short, we must provide not only for the meeting of hygiene needs, but also for the development of enduring satisfiers based on the work of nursing itself and on the elaboration of that work in direct application to client care wherever it is needed—in or out of the hospital.

In the analyses of this study staff, over the period from 1973, a number of encouraging signs point to increased commitment on the part of individuals and of nursing groups to the professionalization of their roles. Growth in the specialty practice groups, development of certification for advanced levels of practice, and encouragement of collaborative role expansion with medicine are all indicators of changing attitudes that are essential to career commitment. There are inadequate indications, however, that our reward system or the general configuration of our utilization patterns for nursing are changing to support and, indeed, to encourage these developments.

What is most needed is a serious examination into the demand side of the manpower equation of nursing, an examination that would look into the development of differential and incremental rewards to foster growth of commitment rather than ignore it—or, in some cases, actually impede development of these rewards.

Long and Disciplined Educational Process

When Abraham Flexner developed his model for the new profession of American medicine, the university system provided the crucial fulcrum for his lever. By lengthening the educational process, by involving basic scientists in the training of medical students, and by emphasizing the importance of both theory and research to the development of a consulting profession, he was able to effect a significant increase in the corpus of medical knowledge in less than 10 years' time.

In 1923 Goldmark and in 1948 Brown [6] sought similar but much more modest changes in the preparation of professional nurses. As a minimum, they wished to establish a collegiate program—at the undergraduate level—that would provide education in the biological and behavioral sciences to supplement the learning of nursing theory and skills. With such a foundation, graduate training could be developed to inculcate research design and methods, additional scientific knowledge, and the expansion of nursing theory and praxis through experimental and rigorous procedures.

The unwillingness of the educational establishment within the hospital schools of nursing to close or transform their programs, coupled with the inability or refusal of state boards to function as advocates and agents for change (as had been the case of medical boards in relation to the Flexner recommendations), doomed the recommendations of the nursing commissions from widespread implementation. No single pattern of nursing education was established, and the majority of the preparatory programs remained stubbornly outside the collegiate mainstream of higher education, impervious to the fact that most minor professions and disciplines were using the collegiate system of the country to upgrade their knowledge base and their claims to competency.

The bifurcation between collegiate and noncollegiate programs was still a source of great frustration and argument in 1966, when the National Commission undertook its work. In the following years, progress has been made toward the resolution of the problem through the reduction of the hospital schools and the opening of collegiate programs. This progress continued at a somewhat reduced pace over the 5 years after 1973. Nevertheless, 25 percent of all the preparatory programs still reside within hospitals, and they admit and graduate about 20 percent of all the beginning registered nurses. Nor is the situation eased by the lack of articulation among many of the 2- and 4-year collegiate programs that shared the responsibility for preparatory education.

The impact of these differences in preparation has serious implications for the profession. In 1970, the Commission staff utilized the Nursing School Environment Inventory to probe the perceptions of students in diploma, associate degree, and baccalaureate programs. Using a striated sample of 283 schools and more than 5000 students, the staff concluded that there were significant differences between the noncollegiate students and both kinds of collegiate students, with the latter reporting higher levels of general esteem, academic enthusiasm, breadth of interest, intrinsic motivation, and encapsulated training (which reflects the clarity of goals in relation to learning experiences). The hospital school students were significantly higher in their perception of extrinsic motivation within the educational setting. In the course of this longitudinal study, our staff, in cooperation with the National Student Nurses' Association, utilized a related survey form that sought to determine how nursing students in the different preparatory programs might perceive an ideal learning environment. A random sample of 600 students was drawn in accordance with current enrollment figures in the three kinds of preparatory programs. Again, significant differences emerged. Collegiate students emphasized the need for theory, research, basic sciences, related arts, and electives much more frequently than did the hospital students. On the other hand, the diploma students were significantly higher than their collegiate counterparts in emphasizing the need for practical applications, involvement with patients, and the desirability of improved goal definition. No differences were to be found between the groups in the areas of importance of scholarship, nursing science, or faculty interaction. In relation to an overall estimate of the quality of their educational experience, the collegiate students rated the excellence of their education at significantly higher levels than did the hospital school students.

The studies in 1970 and in 1977–1978 corroborate each other, but, more important, they emphasize the fact that collegiate and noncollegiate programs essentially develop and socialize their students into different sets and expectations. If one wishes to develop a long and disciplined educational process as a standard for the increased professionalization of nursing, then, it is essential that knowledge be valued for its own sake and that theory and research be recognized as vital components in the enhancement of the nursing armamentarium. From our analyses, collegiate graduates of both 2- and 4-year programs shared comparable attitudes in this regard—differences between the two levels were found, but were not statistically significant. Graduates of the hospital schools of nursing tend to place higher value on the immediate and practical, which reflects the orientation that these institutions have fostered since their very inception. The differences are not a matter of semantics or of mere emphasis; they are of an elemental character that can affect all further learning and applied behavior.

There is certainly room for difference within the preparatory curricula for professional nursing, but to expect that the noncollegiate patterning and emphases can fit into the lengthy and disciplined process that full professions espouse is simply not possible—at least not in terms of the present configuration of the hospital schools of nursing. It is time—past time—for nursing to enter the twentieth century and prepare for the twenty-first. A collegiate pattern of preparatory education is essential to professionalization. Once in place, the matter of articulation between lower- and upper-division programs can be addressed and resolved. Then, and only then, can a true system for preparatory and graduate education be established that can lead to the elaboration of a viable and scientific corpus of knowledge to guide professional practice. Only when all this is accomplished can nursing claim, with rightful assertion, that it is prepared to accept the arduous task of preparing its practitioners for full standing as consulting professionals.

Unique Body of Knowledge and Skill

Closely linked to the concept of disciplined knowledge and learning is the claim to some unique body or configuration of knowledges and skills that sets nursing apart from other practitioner groups—most particularly medicine. It is not necessary that nursing develop an exclusive corpus of lore wholly distinct from those of other disciplines and professions. What is essential is that nursing learn to weave the undergirding sciences and disciplines that support nursing practice into a distinctive combination of elements that make a unique contribution to health care and its delivery. As Scott has pointed out incisively, "Nursing care is the type of care in which multiple factors—biological, psychological, interpersonal, organizational, environmental—converge to produce a given outcome. Areas like this pose a special challenge to researchers" [7]. Nursing research must, by necessity, always contain a goodly amount of interdisciplinary content, but in client care the focus should clearly be on the improvement of nursing intervention.

Early efforts to pursue research in nursing often tended to concern themselves with education and administration. Strauss, for one, argues that this was the natural result of the emphasis of technique over theory in the early hospital training programs and the decision to develop the first educational program for graduate nurses in the confines of Teachers College [8]. Thus, the preparation of both nurses and faculty for schools of nursing was removed from the basic science environment that characterized the growth of medical advancement. More recently, both the emphasis and the content of nursing research have changed. Gortner and others see, in the period since 1970, a growing effort to build a science of nursing practice through systematic inquiry into the effects of nursing intervention, analysis of patient needs, and related investigations into the health behavior of people which can affect or be affected by nursing intervention [9].

In particular, five categories of research have been supported by the federal Division of Nursing over the past several years. These include studies on:

1 Health problems that essentially define the parameters of need for nursing intervention
2 Clinical therapeutics in terms of both procedures and interpersonal aspects of nursing care
3 Analytic and experimental studies on the environments for health care and their relation to effectiveness and efficiency of intervention
4 Development of methodologies and measurement tools for the assessment of quality in nursing care
5 Inquiry into the transference of research findings into the praxis of nursing for the improvement of patient care on broader and more rapid bases

These categories represent the development of a true focus for professional inquiry into nursing practice that extends the beginnings reported on in *An Abstract for Action* and *From Abstract into Action*. These areas of inquiry have been paralleled by a dramatic increase in federal support for nursing research and research training over the past decade. Unfortunately, there are two residual problems that will long continue to limit progress toward an authoritative body of knowledge to guide the development of nursing practice. The first of these is the lack of qualified researchers; the second is the lack of support outside the federal government for the funding of inquiry into nursing intervention.

Largely as the result of the disarray in the preparatory paths to nursing education, there has long been a deficit in the graduate education of nurses—most particularly at the doctoral level, which is essentially the point in American higher education at which research skills and competencies are honed. Of the almost 2000 registered nurses in this country who have earned doctorates, most received their degrees in related professional fields, such as education, administration, or the basic sciences. Between 1974 and 1978, the period of particular interest for this longitudinal survey, doctoral enrollments in schools of nursing increased from 482 to 789. The number of universities offering doctoral training in nursing climbed to 21, but the number of graduations has shown a pattern of decline from a high mark of 74 graduations in 1975 to a figure of 53 in 1978. These figures are simply inadequate to the task of developing the information base necessary to improve professional practice in nursing. Additional graduates are continuing to come out of doctoral programs in related disciplines, but there is no evidence that we can develop that "critical mass" of rigorous researchers needed to determine the impact and the enhancement of nursing practice.

Likewise, the somewhat tentative efforts over the past several years to attract nonfederal dollars into the support of nursing research have not been crowned with signal success. Yet, over this same period of time, a considerable number of approved research proposals sat as a backlog in the files of the Division of Nursing. Complete reliance on federal dollars runs both the risk of abrupt shifts in government policy and priorities and the danger of neglecting the foundations, corporations, and private philanthropists who need to be more aware of the problems and the promises of inquiry into nursing practice. Small but important progress has been made in this area of professionalization since 1973.

Discretionary Authority and Judgment

One of the reported reasons for withdrawal from nursing portrayed in the UPI survey was the feeling of limitation placed on nursing role performance by peers, physicians, and administrators. Perhaps no other area of professional criteria had, however, been altered so dramatically between 1973 and 1978 than had that dealing with discretionary authority and judgment. The growth of collaborative decision making between medicine and nursing as exemplified in the national and statewide joint practice committees, followed by the modification of state practice acts and statutory definitions, significantly expanded the scope of discretion and action in nursing practice.

Although there are and will be continuing disagreements over the independent versus the interdependent role of nurse clinicians and over the ultimate nature of physician supervision, there is indisputable evidence that increased responsibility by nurses in clinical settings has been welcomed for the most part by physicians and, indeed, has been defended and supported in the face of complaint and criticism. This effort must be followed up by professional nursing, particularly the specialty practice groups, to ensure that advanced practitioners are truly competent and that adequate measures are set up to measure and certify clinical specialists and to provide continuing learning experiences that will ensure the maintenance of acquired skills.

In some ways, this study staff feels medicine and nursing, through the joint practice committees and practice acts, have made a contract, almost an affirmation of faith, that nursing will continue and expand its efforts to provide clinical practitioners and leaders with skills and competencies far beyond the normative level of those measures as assessed today. This agreement is not as unusual as it may sound. Physicians recognize that the cutting edge of professionalism is at the point of practice. It is here that research questions are formulated, new interventions delineated, and the requirements for education elaborated. Thus, by providing for increased scope of practice in nursing even before the long and disciplined educational process is in place and before research has carefully delineated a unique pattern of nursing care behaviors, medical and nurse practitioners have provided the environment for incubation and growth.

Progress in clinical authority and judgment has been made. There is a need for nursing to pursue other areas of independence and responsibility. In terms of policy making and planning, nursing made strides over the 5 years but still is underrepresented on many critical groups out of all proportion to its size and potential contribution to health care delivery. Also, the traditional arrangement of organized health care facilities has placed nurses in a subordinate position to administrators as well as physicians. The growing collaboration in clinical areas between medicine and nursing should be accompanied by a companion examination of nurse-administrator functions and relations.

Finally, there is the area of intraprofessional authority. Nursing still experiences periodic upsets in the competitive struggle for organizational ascendancy. Competition more than cooperation is the modus vivendi among the associations and groups that speak for nursing. A more authoritative approach, based on coalescence, would go a long way toward securing attainment of professional standards in all those areas we have described. When nursing speaks for *all* nursing, then, the public and the significant others will listen; but when the voice of nursing is discordant and diffused, everyone will feel free to listen selectively and heedlessly—and no one will really listen.

Cohesive Professional Organization

Implicit in the statement on discretionary authority is the concern of this study staff for the development of a collaborative approach to the analysis of issues and to the enunciation, as much as possible, of a clear, thoughtful, and unified nursing position. In 1970, the National Commission noted with regret that the majority of nurses were not affiliated with any national organization or association and that this lack of participation meant that any critic could attack any nursing position on the basis that it was not representative of the viewpoint held by other nurses—the latter frequently unidentified.

The fragmentation that begins in nursing at the preparatory education level culminates in the fact that fewer than one out of five nurses belongs to any organization that attempts to speak for nursing at the national level. By far the largest single professional body is the American Nurses' Association, but it has a membership only slightly in excess of 200,000. Nurse specialty practice groups have shown the greatest rate of growth over the period of this longitudinal study, and they now have a combined membership of well over 100,000. Because of its membership structure, the National League for Nursing has only a few thousand individual nurse members, but its influence through accreditation and agency activities is very significant. Whether the Federation of Nursing Specialty Organizations and The American Nurses' Association, as well as other efforts to achieve unity and collaboration, will emerge as a vehicle for concerted, authoritative voices for nursing remains very much to be seen.

In comparison with 1973, today there is even more contradictory evidence on the development of a cohesive professional organization. No pronounced growth has taken place with the ANA, and its state nurses' association reports an almost steady membership condition, with increases in one state offset by declines in another. Attempts at collaborative development of certification procedures between the ANA and specialty practice groups have not materialized successfully, and the probability is gathering that new issues, such as accreditation and credentialing, will serve to weaken rather than to cement relationships.

What is terribly needed for the professionalization of nursing is a new birth of leadership, individual and organizational, that can conceive of ways to unite the more than 20 associations that currently draw their membership from nurses. There should be ample acceptance of specific goals and programmatic diversity, but there must, conceivably, be a singularly overriding agreement on such issues as commitment, disciplined educational process, research into the knowledge base, and other professional standards. If these do not exist as a common platform for professional attainment, then their accomplishment is an impossibility and nursing will never attain true status as a principal among the consulting health professions.

Nursing could be considered as the slumbering giant of all American occupations. By this staff's reckoning, there will be, by the end of 1980, more than 2 million persons who will have at some time earned their registered nurse license. More than three-quarters of those will likely retain their license, even though many will not be employed in nursing. Those numbers alone, if they worked in concert, could elect a national president and replace a congress; is it too much to suggest that they work together to construct a professional House of Nursing that can effectively address the full professionalization of their practice for the mutual benefit of themselves and the American public?

Effective and dynamic leadership could accomplish that end given reasonable support through followership. Unfortunately, this study staff could not find any general urgency among the associations and organizations. Many have a sense of some need for greater cooperation, but few are willing to sacrifice the least part of self-determination or territory. Perhaps a presidential veto is the only stimulus to which nursing groups can respond as one. For the marshaling of effective efforts toward professionalization, however, we must have a continuous developmental plan, and it must involve proactive elements as well as those that are reactive. Nursing must profess what it wants and likes—not just what it shuns and dislikes. And, most important of all, it must gather consensus within its own ranks on the basic elements and distinguishing marks of professionalism. If it does that, it can attain the status of a profession; if it does not, then it does not merit that consideration. If the latter proves to be the case, it follows that those who value professionalism should ponder seriously the value of establishing their own professional body and leave nursing to the ambiguous provinces that it currently occupies.

Acknowledged Social Worth

One of the paradoxes long apparent in the perception of American nursing is that there is a strong underpinning of public support and admiration for the profession, but much of the substance of that support is based on a conception of nursing as a "soft" discipline with an ability to provide "tender, loving care" and not much else. The public image of nursing up to 1973 was largely based on the vocational and occupational perceptions of earlier generations, unencumbered by a recognition of the changes that were taking place particularly in the late sixties and early seventies —changes that have continued at a somewhat accelerated pace over the 5 years up to 1978.

This public image constitutes a problem for the further professionalization of nursing. Most Americans like what they think nursing is; most Americans probably fail to understand how it has already changed; few Americans are apt to comprehend what nursing can become in a few short years if it mobilizes its educational and practice patterns into a true professional framework. It is essential that nursing expand the interaction it has initiated with consumer groups and interdisciplinary bodies so as to lay its developmental story before the public. This is not a new insight at all. Nursing more than any other health occupation has invited the scrutiny and participation of outside elements. It is time for this involvement in public participation to be emphasized and for the profession to seek not only advice and counsel but also active support in its efforts to professionalize.

In the conduct of its site visits and interviews, this study staff was uniformly impressed with the extent of public appreciation of nursing's potential in direct proportion to its understanding of the developmental processes and efforts to improve client care. There is a base of recognition and approval that only awaits nursing's call. But there must be a definitive plan for action by the profession to give direction and acceleration to any movement toward greater professionalization.

PROFESSIONAL STATUS AND POWER

As a concomitant to the concept of achieving certain general standards of professionalization it is essential for any occupation that aspires to full professional recognition to understand the essentials of the legal and organizational processes that clearly demarcate a profession from another type of vocational grouping. In an effort to develop a conceptual scheme by which nursing might judge its present position and its most proximate goals, the study staff conceived the graphic presentation displayed in Figure 2–4. On the horizontal axis are those stages that represent increasing elements in the self-regulation of a profession; on the vertical axis are those elements that establish the degree of autonomy accorded a group largely by its acceptance as an altruistic body. To put it another way, on the horizontal axis we assess the extent to which public regulation is either conducted in a manner to support the profession or is, essentially, deeded to the profession for its own administration. In the same context, the vertical axis represents areas in which private regulation is customary and public action is initiated essentially at the volition of the professional group itself.

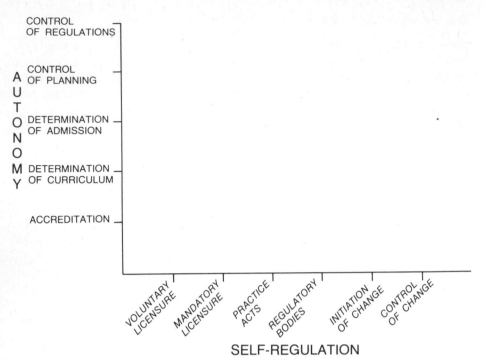

Figure 2–4   Representation of professional status and power.

On the horizontal axis, for example, voluntary licensure is a process by which one may apply for a license or registration to conduct any sort of professional activity. Mandatory licensure is more demanding in the sense that any individual who meets the specifications for licensure may be designated a practitioner by title, but no one who is unlicensed may use that particular title as a generic term to describe his or her intervention. Thus, in a state with voluntary licensure for nurses, anyone could advertise herself as a nurse, but only one who had passed the licensure test could use the title *registered nurse.* In the case of mandatory licensure, no one except those who are licensed may call herself a nurse. Proceeding along the axis, we can assess the degree to which any professional group is involved in the formulation of practice acts and the extent to which it is represented in the composition of regulatory boards, in the initiation of statutory change, and in the control of those changes.

An example may be of help. Medicine, after Flexner, clearly established the principle of mandatory licensure. No one may legally bill himself as a physician without having complied with the requirements of the state in which he practices. Moreover, the practice acts of the several states clearly delimit the extent of medical practice, and these acts are quite generally formulated by physicians who serve as experts and consultants on the provisions of such regulations. In most instances, the regulatory body, or medical board, is largely if not entirely composed of physicians, and this body either initiates statutory change or is consulted in the event that some proposal is generated from the outside. In the last analysis, however, the regulatory body is essentially charged with the control of change, so that its interpretation and guidelines strongly influence the impact and direction of initiatives. In the truest sense, medicine, in most states, is self-regulated, and the lay public has ceded to the profession those powers that might be described as the police powers for the control of medical practice.

In examining the vertical axis, we see related but somewhat divergent forms of control. Accreditation has long been seen as a joint venture between state and national associations, with the major verification of competency coming from the discipline or profession involved. Likewise, state agencies have been reluctant to intrude into the determination of curriculum (with the possible exception of professional education, which is seen as a logical extension of the state's mandate to provide for public education). Admission standards, before the era of affirmative action and minority rights, were largely reserved to the institution without question, as was the control of local planning for the initiation of new programs, the phasing out of others, and the allocation of resources among the existing. Finally, the control and determination of regulations for certification, recertification, and various forms of advanced recognition were frequently delegated to the profession or its educational institutions.

To use the example of medicine again, accreditation was bestowed on committees composed of representatives from the American Medical Association and the American Association of Medical Colleges. State agencies might play a part, but professional acceptance and professional mobility required an imprimatur from the relevant associations. The curriculum was determined entirely by the medical faculty using guidelines from the accrediting associations, although in recent years both federal and state governments have attempted to mandate, cajole, or influence by funding the development of new curricular emphases—most particularly that of family medicine. Admissions were once sacrosanct, but are increasingly subject to judicial review and appeal—and reappeal. Control of institutional planning is subject, in part, to pressures from state and federal governments to increase class size or to establish new medical colleges, but the control of specialization and advanced certification is essentially reserved to medicine through its boards and institutions.

In short, the profession of medicine in 1960 had almost total control over the elements of both self-regulation and autonomy as here defined. Their history, more recently, has been one of challenge and encroachment by some state and federal agencies with the intent to limit either the autonomy or the self-regulation of the profession.

In marked contrast to the reverse movement in medicine, nursing since 1973 has largely gravitated toward a position of increased power, albeit in large part because it was operating from a level of deprivation. When the National Commission undertook its study of American nursing, eight states still practiced voluntary licensure for registered nursing. Practice acts were restrictive; regulatory bodies, even when composed of nurses only, were sharply divided on matters of education and professional practice. The initiation and control of change were outside the jurisdiction of the profession. Accreditation and the control of the curriculum (so long as it was traditional) were not problematic, but the determination of admission and the control of planning were largely a function of the assessed nursing shortage within the state, and there was no professional control or regulation beyond the preparatory level.

Since 1973, nursing has asserted and won its increasing right to self-regulation and autonomy. It has moved successfully toward increased mandatory licensure; it has successfully enlarged the scope of practice acts in a majority of the states; and it has had some impact on the decisions and considerations of regulatory bodies. If it has not controlled change, it has more often than not been the advocate of change in licensure and in practice definitions. It has controlled accreditation, curriculum, and determination of admissions (largely through its past record of involvement in minority access). It has been involved in both the control of planning and the control of regulations and certification for advanced levels of practice.

Indeed, in contrast to some of the growing pressures on medicine to conform and to accept greater outside regulation, the attitude toward nursing has been to allow it more freedom to assert its own formulas for professional advancement. The prime difficulty we see is the inability of nursing to determine one overall goal for each factor in the continuum of professionalization. When nursing secures the right of program control, for example, it is still left with a division between proponents of collegiate education and the defenders of the noncollegiate sequence. Occasionally, by default, the resolution of these viewpoints has been left to those outside the profession. Every instance of this is evidence of the inability of nursing to govern and control itself.

Sometime before the end of this century, nursing must face up to the fact that it is, in essential characteristics, its own worst enemy. It can be its own best friend, but it must demonstrate its ability to develop consensus, professional priorities, and assertive action to carry out its professed ambitions.

A COMMENTARY ON PROFESSIONALISM

Some years ago, a distinguished sociologist who was a committed friend of nursing observed that nurses had a distinct predilection for defining goals without any concern for the routes or steps to achieve them. Since 1967, some members of this study staff have heard and read the protestations of nursing for professionalization. This goal is commendable and honorable. It can, however, be achieved only by the processes that have characterized every other claim to full professionalism. It cannot be achieved by a part-time group of functionaries, or by a confused and confusing educational melange. It cannot be realized without research and a unique body of knowledge and skill. Nor can it be realized by the abdication of authority and responsibility or by the absence of internal consensus.

Perhaps the clearest call to an examination of ends and means is afforded in the humorous but insightful words of Scott when he says, "If you still insist on harboring the question of the status of nursing, let me help you to this extent . . . 'Is she or isn't she?' is best decided by asking, 'Does she or doesn't she?'"[10] Professionals are as professionals do. In retrospect, nursing has become more professional since

1973, but on no single dimension can it clearly and forcefully prove its independent right to autonomy or self-regulation. Moreover, there are elements within nursing that have fought almost every act of increased responsibility or heightened level of practice. In a fast-shortening time, nursing must resolve its own ambiguities before it can assert its right to self-determination. The prognosis is good, but the patient is subject to improbable, destructive impulses.

It will be good for the health care consumers of America if nursing takes on the responsibility incumbent on a true profession. We can support, we can encourage, but no one can do for nursing what it must do for itself. The goals are evident; the pathways clearly demarcated. Success or failure, first and foremost, lies in the nurses, their organizations, and their leaders.

REFERENCES

1 Ethline Mais, "Nursing Professionalization in America," unpublished position paper, Center for Educational Administration and Human Development, The University of Rochester, Rochester, N.Y., 1979.
2 *NJPC Bulletin,* vol. 4, no. 2, December 1978, pp. 10–11.
3 Abraham Flexner, *Medical Education in the United States and Canada,* D. B. Updike, the Merrymount Press, Boston, 1960.
4 Josephine Goldmark, *Nursing and Nursing Education in the United States,* The Macmillan Co., New York, 1923.
5 Patricia McCormack, "Shortage of Nurses, a National Problem," *Democrat and Chronicle,* Rochester, N.Y., September 23, 1979, pp. 19a–21a.
6 Esther Lucile Brown, *Nursing for the Future,* Russell Sage Foundation, New York, 1948.
7 W. Richard Scott, "Professional Work and Professional Power: Some Implications for Nursing," unpublished paper, Rush University, Chicago, March 1976, p. 11.
8 Anselm Strauss, "The Structure and Ideology of American Nursing: An Interpretation," in Fred Davis (ed.), *The Nursing Profession: Five Sociological Essays,* John Wiley & Sons, New York, 1966.
9 Susan R. Gortner, Doris Bloch, and Thomas P. Phillips, "Contributions of Nursing Research to Patient Care," *Journal of Nursing Administration,* March–April 1976, pp. 22–28.
10 Scott, op. cit., p. 3.

Chapter 3

Characteristics, Concepts, and Scope of Nursing Practice

No effort to understand the dynamics of change in nursing can afford to ignore the societal trends that have so deeply affected our understanding of health care and its delivery. Technological change has been a common phenomenon in medicine and in health treatment since the Flexnerian emphases on theory and research pushed back the frontiers of knowledge. More recently, however, economic pressures and political changes have been more determinative of care allocation and delivery than ever before. It is not simply a matter of difference in degree, but rather an essential change in kind.

As indicated in Figure 3–1, social and cultural forces have replaced advances in medical science as forcing trends in the decision making on our health system. Health treatment, indeed health maintenance and preventive care, are seen as rights the professional must provide, and the pressure continues to mount for a comprehensive national health care system that will encompass all these demands. In September of 1979, President Carter chided Senator Kennedy for not having had a bill for national health insurance pass the Congress and promised that he would obtain such a measure and sign it. The opposition party has differed largely in terms of the extent to which private third-party payers might be involved along with public agencies, and the American Medical Association (AMA) has even advanced its own proposals for a form of national health coverage.

- Social and Cultural Change

- Advances in Medical Science

- Changed Economics of Health

Figure 3-1 Trends in American health care and delivery, 1979.

Politically aware pressure groups ranging from the Gray Panthers to the groups advocating abortion availability for minors, along with formidable trade unions and minority action blocks, have targeted national health insurance as a top priority, and the only question after what specific form it shall take is how we are to carry it off. The answer is, of course, unknown, but one of the major contributors to a solution has got to be a vastly upgraded contingent of nurse practitioners functioning with vigor in an expanded scope of practice that embodies altered concepts on the requirements for and limitations of nurse role behavior.

In this regard, the *Report of the Secretary's Committee to Study Extended Roles for Nurses* [1], published in 1971, was prophetic in its insistence not only on an expansion of the nursing role—which some might have regarded as simply doing a bit more of the same—but also on the development of whole new practice capabilities in primary care, acute treatment, and long-term functions for the chronically ill and injured. With the establishment of the National Joint Practice Commission (NJPC) in the same year, organized medicine and nursing sought to describe and develop new collaborative approaches to care which would mean role change in both professions. The progress they have achieved is discussed at length in Chapter 4 of this report.

From their planning and demonstration projects, however, and from the advances in medical science, it is increasingly clear that comprehensive health care is far broader than the one-time view that held the physician to be the single individual ultimately responsible for total patient treatment. In fact, we now understand care to be something much greater than collaboration between medicine and nursing or any other formal simplistic arrangement. We have not replaced Ptolemaic formulations with those of a Copernicus and simply reordered the health care universe around another central figure. What we have developed is a nonconcentric pattern in which health care practitioners and specialists essentially move in and out—we hope in rational rather than random patterns—depending on the needs of the patient.

In this model, a schematic diagram of one condition of which is indicated in Figure 3-2, patients, as well as the professional practitioners, play a lead role and perhaps also must assume greater responsibility than they have felt in the past, when they could remain quite passive and place the burden of care on others. Care becomes a multivariate interaction among physicians, nurses, therapists, family, and self. In complex surgical procedures, teams of 40 or 60 professionals may be involved, whereas in a community health maintenance organization, an individual subscriber may have his or her own physician and nurse and a choice of using either

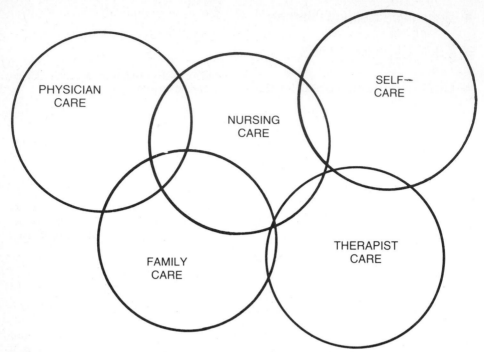

Figure 3–2   Identity and interdependence of functions in an emergent pattern of health care delivery.

or both depending on the situation—with the understanding that referral will be made to any specialist as needed.

This emergent pattern of practitioner relationships would be necessary if for no other reason than to respond to massive consumer demands. Even without the addition of national health insurance, it is estimated that private health insurers, including the Blue Cross and Blue Shield plans, cover as many as 177 million Americans for hospital expenses, with up to 147 million people protected by major medical plans that offer insurance against catastrophic expenses. Additional millions of individuals are covered through Medicare and Medicaid, leaving, as indicated in Figure 3–3, approximately 15 to 18 million uninsured according to 1978 estimates of the Department of Health, Education, and Welfare. Essentially, then, we largely have a form of prepaid national health plan in existence for most Americans; federal health insurance will blanket in those who now are uninsured and expand the coverage of others. Whether demand will really soar, however, in the event of national health insurance is debatable—largely because of the extensive system of coverage we have already set in place.

Another reason, however, for the reconfiguration of the patterning for health care delivery is the probable change in the *nature* of the demand for health services apart from the *level* of that demand. In recent years, the request of the consumer is no longer merely one for cure, but for health. Health maintenance, preventive intervention, and widespread lay interest in exercise, weight reduction, and health

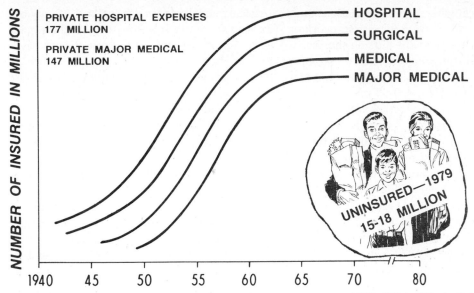

Figure 3–3   Schematic representation of health insurance coverage, 1979. *(Original illustration based on information generally available from HEW, NLN, ANA, and AHA.)*

regimens have been notably on the increase. This public awareness not only provides hope that a national health insurance system can be a workable concept, but it also materially challenges the characteristics and scope of practice that have been traditional in a profession such as nursing. The situation calls for new practitioner roles and for innovative approaches to the delivery of care.

THE CLIMATE OF NURSING CARE

In 1970, the National Commission reported that the climate of nursing practice was greatly affected by the impression of perpetual shortages, by an impoverished work environment, and by a generalized misunderstanding of the role of the nurse in a developing health care system. Today, we have much greater insight into these phenomena, and it is essential that the consumer public become aware of the ferment that is taking place in relation to the climate of nursing care.

Climate of Nursing Shortage

In Chapter 2, we treated the problem of retention in nursing and indicated that there would be no talk of a nursing shortage at all if we were to maintain the contribution of only a portion of those nurses who leave the profession—or at least leave employment within the profession. In September of 1979, the president of the American Nurses' Association (ANA), in response to a query from United Press International, estimated that the current "shortage" of nurses in the United States ran between 45,000 and 60,000 [2]. In the very same discussion, it was pointed out that over 395,000 nurses were working part time and an additional 420,000 were not working at all! It is this incredible paradox that constantly impacts on any discussion of nursing roles and functions and that renders understanding so difficult. If only one out of every five nurses working part time shifted to full time, the numbers game that we call a nursing shortage would disappear. Likewise, if one out of every seven inactive nurses was to take up practice, there would be no shortage to report.

There is much more at stake here, however, than the refutation of an absurd assertion. A brief review of nursing manpower figures, both projections of need and analyses of actual activity, may be useful in assessing our directions for the future. In Figure 3–4 there is displayed the relationship our Commission observed between a variety of estimates of the future nursing manpower and the actual number of prepared nurses through 1969. Based on the fact that actual nursing manpower figures almost always equaled or exceeded even the most generous projections of need, our staff projected that the actual nursing manpower would rise above the most generous assessment of the surgeon general's 1968 projection for the decade ahead. As indicated in Figure 3–5, this rise was accomplished in spectacular fashion largely because of an 80 percent increase in graduations from preparatory nursing programs between 1970 and 1976. The rate of growth has leveled off more recently, and we may actually experience a drop in graduations on a year-to-year basis, but this drop

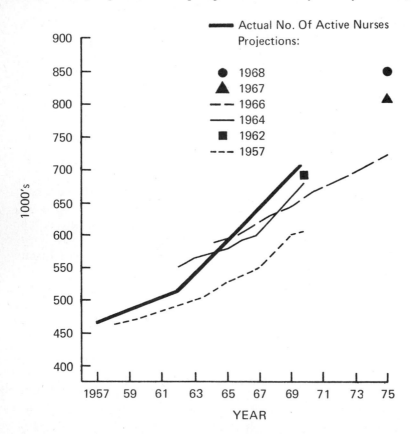

Figure 3–4   Actual number of nurses in relationship to projected numbers, 1957–1975.

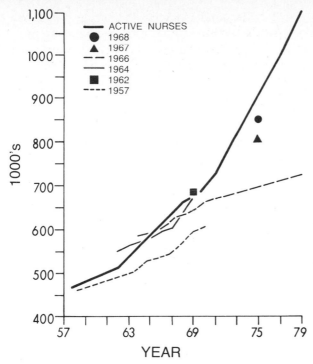

Figure 3–5   Actual number of nurses in relationship to projected numbers, 1957–1979.

will be a function as much of declining high school and college enrollments as of any facet of nursing education.

The point is simply that American nursing has girded itself to respond to calls for more and more students and for more and more graduates. This capability not only meets the goals set by the "experts" in health manpower planning, but assumes significant proportions in the real world of health care. For example, in Figure 3–6, we can compare the trends in nurse-to-population ratios from before the inquiry of the National Commission to the present. Not only have we increased the supply of nurses dramatically, but in terms of relationship to population we have come from about 319 nurses per 100,000 to 500 nurses per 100,000 population.

A summary of the growth of the nurse-to-population ratio at 2-year intervals is presented in Figure 3–7. This growth is particularly interesting when one considers that a composite of projections in 1966 indicated that all health requirements in this country would be met when a ratio of 350 nurses per 100,000 could be attained. This figure was actually exceeded in the year that *An Abstract for Action* appeared, but, in 1979, we continue to hear the same assertions of a nursing shortage after we have exceeded that magic figure by a full 43 percent. It would appear that much of the nursing shortage is a Parkinsonian phantasm in which "need" continually rises to swallow up any increase in supply with no indication that we are any closer to a definitive solution of the problems of nursing manpower.

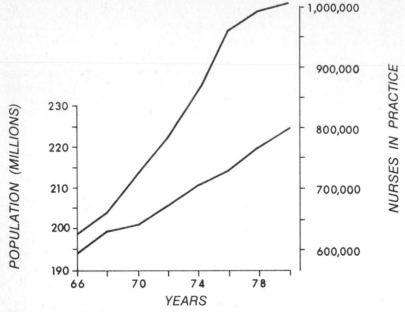

Figure 3–6   Trends in nurse-to-population ratios, 1966–1979.

If we can accept the simple premise that the nursing shortage is a complex phenomenon that cannot be solved merely by the production of ever and ever greater numbers of new graduates, and if we can agree that there is something woefully lacking in our ability to retain these individuals in the practice of their profession, we will have come a long way toward the realization that new concepts and characteristics of nursing roles are essential not only to the improvement of health care but also to the stabilization of our entire system for health care delivery.

Work Environment and Role Misunderstanding

Because these aspects of the current nursing climate in America are treated in detail in Chapters 4 and 6, it would be redundant to entertain them at length here. Suffice it to say that the milieu of the nursing work environment, including its reward

NURSES PER 100,000 POPULATION

1966	----------------------	319
1968	----------------------	335
1970	----------------------	356
1972	----------------------	376
1974	----------------------	407
1976	----------------------	449
1978	----------------------	478
1980	----------------------	500

Figure 3–7   Summary review of nurse-to-population ratios, 1966–1980. *(Original illustration based on information generally available from HEW, ANA, NLN, AHA, etc.)*

systems and intrinsic satisfactions, is capable of sending 50 percent of our graduate nurses fleeing from any form of active involvement in the practice of the profession for which they were prepared. Any other profession or employer group for that profession would consider this condition an unmitigated disaster. It is a commentary on the climate of nursing that one of the proposals for solving the nursing shortage reported in the United Press International feature story in the fall of 1979 was for a return to the establishment of schools of nursing in most hospitals [3]. There was not a single indication that the split in nursing education between collegiate and noncollegiate tracks is one of the contributors to the impoverished work environment of nursing—and to the withdrawal of disillusioned individuals who feel they have been "used" in the manipulation of people and resources to maintain a divided and depressed system at the expense of those who seek to keep it operable.

Talleyrand had in mind the French Bourbons when he declared, "They never learn anything from experience, nor do they ever forget." He might, however, have just as well been speaking of hospital administrators who see the return of hospital schools as a solution to the nursing shortage. Adequate compensation levels, incremental increases for exhibited excellence in clinical practice, promotion around patient care rather than into administration, and a host of other real changes in the work environment of nurses are essential to halt the retreat of qualified practitioners from what is often a no-win situation.

In Chapter 4, there is documentation of the many positive changes that have taken place—largely in connection with the joint development of collaborative goals between medicine and nursing since 1973. This direction must be continued and must increasingly involve administrators and other health practitioners so that communications and understanding will facilitate the elaboration of new roles and relationships.

Progress has been made since 1973 in terms of both work environment and role understanding in nursing, but the deficits of the past decades cannot be made up in a few short years—nor can there be any expectation of reaching a point of permanent equilibrium. One of the realities of the emergent health care system is that change will be a primary characteristic and that nursing will be as subject to alteration as any other agency in the unfolding of the dynamics of that new pattern. Administrators and directors of nursing service who wish for a return to the former predictability of nursing are not obsolescent in terms of the emergent health care system—they are obsolete.

Toward a New Climate for Nursing

In 1970, it was apparent to the National Commission that American nursing had long made its contributions to health care in this country largely in spite, rather than because, of the traditional organizational arrangements and personnel policies of our health care facilities. Nurses were used essentially as interchangeable parts in the system; they were expected to function as fully experienced and qualified professionals on the day after their graduation although no one questioned the need for a graduate physician to continue his training through an internship and even a residency period. Though it was not included in the nursing curriculum, registered nurses were expected to supervise and train auxiliary personnel to perform functions that should have been reserved to the repertoire of professional nursing—and were then held responsible for the safe and effective conduct of such procedures even though they were not personally carrying them out. Nurses were expected to provide the middle management of the health care facility and were actually paid more to abstain from practice than to engage in patient care.

The relationship between nursing and medicine—although there have always been strong ties at the individual and small group level—often institutionally assumed the characteristics of an adversary meeting. Many physicians not only arrogated to themselves the right to define the nursing role and to unilaterally establish the ground rules for cooperation, but also became the authorities on how and where nursing education should be conducted. (Exactly where the knowledge about nursing education was formulated in the training of either physicians or hospital administrators is only one of the small mysteries in the historical development of nursing.) As a result, nursing found itself constantly on the defensive and, predictably, often reacted in an unpredictable fashion.

Out of a climate of frustration, mistrust, and hostility, there is emerging a new professional harmony between nursing and medicine first and, more recently, between nursing and health administration. Exploration of new initiatives and relationships must be permitted and each profession must perform those roles that are proper and most productive and divest those that are historic accidents or vestiges of earlier, unplanned transfers of activity and responsibility. In all this, if nursing is treated as an intelligent and equal partner in the planning, this study staff is confident that improved configurations will emerge that will be more effective and efficient than our present nonsystem. We hope the models being developed by the National Joint Practice Commission (NJPC) for physician-nurse-administrator collaboration in primary hospital care will be a guide that will facilitate general movement throughout our health care facilities [4]. It is very much needed.

CONCEPTS OF NURSING PRACTICE

In its report on American nursing in 1970, the National Commission described three stages in the public's concept of nursing practice that constitute an essential background for any discussion of new role expectations and practice behaviors. It is, perhaps, worthwhile to review those stages in summary fashion in order to better understand not only the need for change, but also the directions that change should emphasize. The stages proposed in *An Abstract for Action* included the vocational concept of American nursing, the occupational concept, and the beginning professional concept of nursing practice.

The Vocational Concept of Practice

For a long period of time, the public view of nursing was largely vague and indistinct —though frequently warm and supportive. The nurse was perceived as essentially bound up within the environment of the hospital (or, occasionally, the public health clinic). She provided care for the patient and some form of administrative service to the institution through the supervision of other workers. There was no perceived overlap between the professional activities of the physician and the ministrations of the nurse although she followed his orders in carrying out certain procedures (see Figure 3–8).

The vocational concept included an understanding that some training was necessary to prepare the nurse for her job, but this training had no great intellectual content and was largely what married women learned experientially through family care and child rearing. It would be necessary to teach a student these things because a nurse, of course, was an unmarried female who served in this occupation only until she married and began a family of her own.

Granted this description is deliberately overdrawn, but some of these character-izations developed an enduring quality that was hard to transform. The depiction of nursing as a female occupation, the clear separation of medical and nursing roles, the boundaries that clearly contained nurses within institutions, and the general feeling that nursing was essentially a surrogate role that could be provided by a wife or mother in a home setting all combined to develop a concept of a useful vocation, but little more.

The attractiveness of such work must be attributed in great part to the lack of alternatives that women faced before and after the turn of the century. By and large,

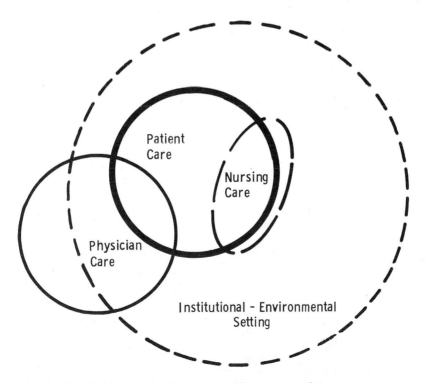

Figure 3–8   Model of the public view of nursing as a vocation.

nursing and school teaching were the only accepted outlets apart from clerical, clerking, or factory types of employment. If it had limited horizons, the girls who entered its ranks likely had no thought of nursing as a career. If it had limitations, so did any other available type of paid employment. At least nursing had the personal, intrinsic satisfactions of caring for people in need and knowing that, in some ways, you were helping them. Indeed, patients and their families responded with warmth and gratitude.

The Occupational Concept of Practice

As the training schools for nursing emerged, with lengthened curriculums and up to 3 years of student learning, the vocational concept of practice receded and was replaced by a more complicated view of nursing as an occupation (see Figure 3–9). The nursing role was now seen as a working ability to perform any one of hundreds of procedures or care tasks that now encompassed a majority of the therapeutic experiences a patient would receive in a hospital or clinic. The physician would write or orally deliver orders and instructions, but the bulk of these would be administered and followed by the nurse.

Nursing practice was seen to overlap in part with the work of the physician, but this was assumed to be in noncritical areas in which the practitioner present would, perhaps, take the pulse or temperature as the occasion demanded. In more complex matters, the physician worked alone or as the supervisor of the nurse who

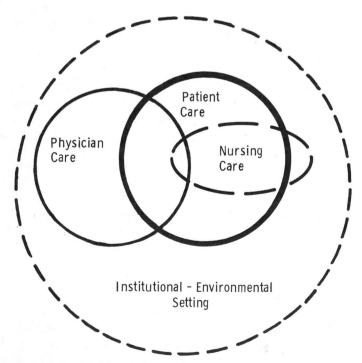

Figure 3–9   Model of the occupational view of nursing practice.

was aiding him in the treatment or operation. Nurses continued to do other things. They supervised other aides and orderlies, they performed administrative tasks, and they provided clinical instruction for the students from the hospital training school. Nevertheless, they were not perceived as professionals because they did not engage in independent practice nor did they make independent decisions. Even when nurses acted in the absence of physicians, there was the ceremonial act of "signing off," which meant that the physician officially assumed professional responsibility for the delegated tasks performed by the nurse.

Unfortunately, this occupational view of nursing did acknowledge the enlarged variety of tasks and procedures that the individual nurse conducted, but was devoid of intellectual content. Nursing was no longer the institutional extension of home health care, but neither was it a part of the physician's armamentarium or practice. Moreover, an increasing number of females in white uniforms began to appear at the bedside, and the public found it more and more difficult to distinguish among nurses, practical nurses, and nurse aides. (So did the physicians, the registered nurses, and the administrators.) Although the occupational view was more support-ive, in general, than the vocational view, it was also subject to increasing confusion and cross-labeling.

Beginning Professional Concepts

Sometime before the Second World War, hastened by the experience of servicemen and -women during the previous war, a new concept began to emerge about nursing. Spurred by the shortage of physicians and the increasing number of nurse college graduates (college education was, after all, a mark of distinction up to the late forties) the lay public began to see the practice of nursing in a new light. Certainly, a nurse was not a substitute for a physician, but she could be a standin and she could exercise judgment and responsibility (see Figure 3–10).

Nurses began to appear more frequently in settings other than the hospital. True, they were employees and not independent practitioners, but they were working in industry, in schools, and in a variety of public health agencies. Increasingly, as the shortage of physicians became pronounced, it was discovered that nurses could exercise judgment and also assume responsibility for the consequences of their decisions. If this concept of nursing did not see a unique role of expertise for the nurse practitioner, it did comprehend the fact that there was a shared domain of knowledge and skill that was larger than had been conceived of during the vocational and occupational stages of nursing role perception.

Somewhere in this period, the public began to accept the distinction between training and education for nurses; there was a body of knowledge, perhaps not unique but nevertheless formidable, which the college-educated nurse had to learn and master. (Unfortunately, all nursing students still were measured by the same licensure examination, and the unwillingness of some nurses and hospital adminis-trators prevented instituting a single collegiate preparation pattern for all nursing students in the general rearrangement of American higher education in the early fifties.)

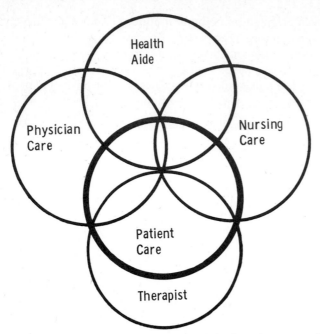

Figure 3–10   Model of the emergent view of nursing as a profession.

Over and above this growing measure of collaborative practice, nursing also asserted its emphasis on psychosocial implications of care, which was not original but was certainly a more pronounced concentration than was exercised by medicine for many years after the Flexnerian explosion. Increasingly, nurses assumed the role of teachers, family consultants, and patient advocates. No one had developed a job description that included these competencies, but once again, practice preceded preparation, and the public responded with approbation and support.

Some administrators, fewer physicians, lamented this growth toward parity if not equality. The greater assumption of responsibility by nurses became a mighty asset in the delivery of care. Individual nurses became more assertive, but the increased knowledge base afforded a new resource to physicians and institutions alike in the accomplishment of patient care. Lost somewhere in this changing perspective was the fact that nurses had begun to assess internal differences and levels of expertise that professionals, let alone laymen, had failed to remark. In this context, the position paper [5] of the American Nurses' Association (ANA) in 1964–1965 represents a real turning point. To accept the principle of college education for all nurses was to accept not only the beginnings of professional nursing, but also the unpredictable consequences of instilling a new, vital force into the process of decision making and policy formulation. Lines were quickly drawn, and the full professionalization concept was challenged by physicians, administrators, and many nurses who felt that they would be excluded from the contemplated actions toward establishing a full profession of nursing.

Toward a Full Profession

Between 1965 and 1970, a full-blown war was waged beneath the surface of American health care institutions and their delivery systems. Administrators, physicians, and some nursing educators extolled the virtues of the hospital training schools and practice environments that had so magnificently provided for the vocational and occupational requirements of nursing service. Apparently unable to comprehend the need of every individual to perceive the opportunity to grow and to extend one's grasp beyond one's reach, these advocates of the status quo argued essentially that formal education in the mainstream of the collegiate institutions was unnecessary for nurses and, in essence, endorsed the decision, made 100 years before, to eschew the full implementation of the Nightingale model for nursing education and service and to substitute therefor an American adaptation that placed pragmatism before disciplined knowledge and compliance before conceptual understanding.

Entirely aside from the concerns of the chief antagonists in this quarrel, events transpired that had immeasurable impact on the later repatterning of the nursing profession. For one, the emergence of the community and junior colleges as an educational force in nursing caught both the hospital school advocates and the baccalaureate champions off guard. Neither saw this development as a fundamental and probably decisive shift toward a collegiate pattern in nursing education. Neither appreciated the fact that associate degree graduates might not have all the capabilities of other collegiate nurses, but shared most of their feelings about theory, research, and full, if eventual, professionalization. Nor did the strident voices of 1965 take into account the perceived need of medicine to acquire new collaborators in the provision of medical and health care to the burgeoning groups that were demanding it not as a benefit but as a right. After a short romance with the possibility of developing a whole new category of health personnel, the physician's assistant, the leaders of American medicine recalled that the nurse had for many years functioned in this role without benefit of title and, moreover, was better educated and trained than most of the alternative functionaries proposed to assume a more responsible role in health care.

Somewhere, too, in this welter of ideas and opinions, the National Commission for the Study of Nursing and Nursing Education (NCSNNE) proposed a new formulation of nursing roles and concepts that might provide a legitimate, rational compromise in the face of anarchy. Committed to the proposition that nursing inherently contained the numbers and the clinical capacity to meet the nation's health needs through a reformulation of its traditional roles, the National Commission proposed that medicine and nursing work in concert to redefine the full professional role of the nurse practitioner while other groups worked to effect a repatterning of education and the development of a career concept that would enhance retention, reduce withdrawal, and prolong the lifespan of a nurse practitioner.

The first requirement of such a conceptualization was the rejection of many of the tenets of the vocational and occupational views of nursing. This rejection was the equivalent of updating one's views of transportation, communications, and marketing, but it was perhaps more poignant because of the empathic, human regard that many held for an outmoded system of patient care that never was as good as we remembered and was likely less helpful than we hoped. The second requirement was the reformulation of a new model of nursing practice that would not only meet the needs of today but also be adaptable to needs still unarticulated. For this purpose, the National Commission devised a new and probabilistic model of nursing practice, which it proposed for the consideration of nursing, medicine, and the public at large.

In place of the largely unidimensional concepts that characterized even the beginnings of a professional acceptance of nursing, the interactive model envisaged three dynamic continua that operate in close relationship to one another and, taken together, can explicate the entire domain of needs for nursing care and expertise. On one plane is the classified set of nursing behaviors ranging from the initial assessment of client condition, through intervention, instruction, back to the assessment of outcomes and results—in short, the rigorous application of scientific method to the direction of nursing activity. On a second plane is an acknowledgment of patient condition. Nowhere in this model do we assume that nursing is a reactive, stimuli-driven set of practitioners. The concept of maintaining wellness and limiting illness is as much a part of the full practice of nursing—or medicine—as is the treatment of acute illness. On the third axis is the concept of environmental setting, which provides for the use of institutionalization, outpatient or clinic care, and home or community settings as proper areas for the enactment of nursing behaviors (see Figure 3–11).

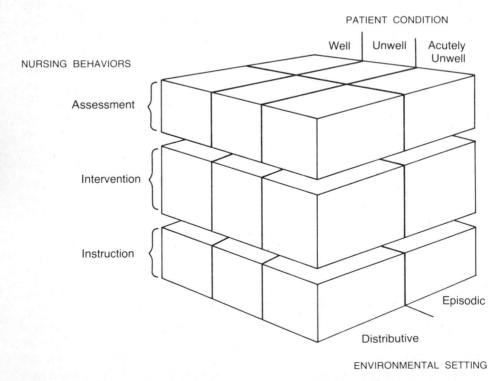

Figure 3–11   Interactive model of an emergent, full profession of nursing.

In contrast to the vocational model of nursing practice, the interactive model emphasizes the independent—or interdependent—role of nurses in determining proper role functions in accordance with client needs and in relationship to selecting the optimum environment for care. This conceptual framework suggests no single locus for nursing practice; it argues for a wide variety of specific capacities in the place of simple skills, and it argues for a relocation of the patient and his or her needs to an elemental position in the decision-making process related to intervention and care. It is not bound to a single institution, a single congruent practicing profession, or a discrete body of clients to be served. Rather it argues for nursing—not nurses —to be prepared for health intervention over a complete kaleidoscope of situations. We say nursing—not nurses—for the simple reason that the interactive model inherently rejects the basic assumption of both the vocational and the occupational concept that nursing is essentially an illness-centered, hospital-focused utility. Within this model, there is room for a wide variety of concentrations and specializations both horizontal—across the range of client care needs (from acute cardiac care, for example, through mild illness to a need for information on the control of hypertension)—and vertically—within a nursing practice (from staff nurse to clinical practitioner to master clinician).

This conceptual scheme not only differentiates practice roles and settings, but also argues for variation in the educational patterning of preparatory and advanced students in order to assure the variety as well as the numbers of nurses needed to implement a full range of client services. It also provides for a commitment and career perspective that includes mobility and incremental increases in responsibility, authority, and recognition. Finally, it can function as a research model for the generation of hypotheses concerning the cognitive, affective, and motor-skill components required for the different combinations of nursing behaviors, client needs, and environmental settings that characterize the subsets of the conceptual framework. In turn, results of experimentation with those hypotheses may give us for the first time precise information on educational and practice patterns related to specific manpower needs in nursing rather than the global kinds of information we attempt to process today. We shall treat this concept in the succeeding section.

PRACTICE CHARACTERISTICS AND NURSE MANPOWER PLANNING

Although concern for nursing manpower goes back to the very beginnings of the training schools which preceded the Nightingale hospital schools, the inclusion of nursing in the formalized apparatus of federal health manpower planning is of more recent vintage. Since 1957, however, there have been frequent projections by the surgeon general's office, the Division of Health Resources, and other groups that have sought to project manpower goals for American nursing. Most of these have resulted in the points and plots portrayed in Figures 3–4 and 3–5. The projections are usually in terms of a round number of so many hundreds of thousands of nurses or so many nurses per 100,000 population, with an implicit preconception that a nurse is a nurse is a nurse. In terms of the interactive model proposed for future role description and expectation, that global form of manpower planning is almost worse than useless.

In 1972, Wood developed a career sequence model for nursing occupations which attempted to add some dimensionality to the manpower planning process [6]. By correlating the exit-level skills that were defined for various stages of nursing education with care requirements specified for different patient-client conditions, she conceptualized five career levels that would provide different combinations of knowledge/skill relationships for the care of patients. As indicated in Figure 3–12, career level 1 would be composed of nurse care providers with a foundation of scientific understanding but with an emphasis on applied skills and nursing arts. This level would be akin to the preparation and exit competencies of the licensed practical or vocational nurse. At career level 4, in contrast, we would expect a much broader understanding of basic science and pathophysiology together with diagnostic skills and an ability to plan therapeutic regimens. This level would be, in current terms, a clinical specialist or master clinician.

Using Wood's divisions and applying our labeling system to the career level concept, we arrive at a projected active nurse population of 2 million for 1980 that would be composed of 500,000 licensed practical nurses (L.P.N.s), 1 million associate degree nurses (A.D.N.s), 300,000 bachelors of nursing (B.S.N.s), 180,000 masters of nursing (M.S.N.s), and 20,000 doctors of nursing (D.S.N.s). We have used these academic titles in relationship to levels in order to express the career sequencing in terms of the emergent collegiate system for nursing education, but we would hasten to add that, for a long time to come, we should append "or equivalent"

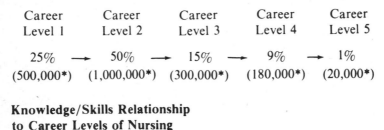

Career Level 1	Career Level 2	Career Level 3	Career Level 4	Career Level 5
25% →	50% →	15% →	9% →	1%
(500,000*)	(1,000,000*)	(300,000*)	(180,000*)	(20,000*)

**Knowledge/Skills Relationship
to Career Levels of Nursing**

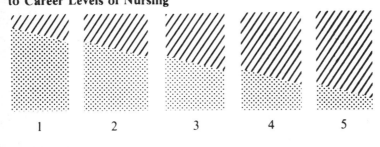

1   2   3   4   5

*Predicated on basis of total nursing population of 2,000,000.   ///// = Knowledge   :::::: = Skills

Figure 3–12   Career sequence for nursing occupations. *(Redrawn from "Career Model for Nurse Practitioners," Lucile A. Wood, director, USDE Grant 8-0627, UCLA, Division of Vocational Education, March 1972. Used with permission.)*

to each category that we have designated. The Wood model is essentially a starting framework, but it begins to reduce our goals for nursing manpower into more meaningful categories and shows us differential surpluses and deficits as we examine the present and consider the future. For example, using the manpower figures compiled by the American Nurses' Association and the National League for Nursing, it would appear that we have more than enough individuals prepared at the first two stages of the Wood schema (using this study staff's labeling pattern), a considerable deficit at stage 3, and dramatic deficits at stages 4 and 5. In other words, our general concern for "nurses per 100,000" has failed to inform us that there are critical imbalances within the figures and that we have surpluses in some areas and critical shortages in others.

The Wood approach, useful as it is, however, is still only a two-dimensional presentation. It should be recognized not only as one of the first empirical attempts to describe and to evaluate related levels of nursing practice, but also as one of the first efforts to develop a career model that would facilitate upward mobility for nurse graduates by relating the learnings at one stage to the required competencies for each succeeding stage. Its influence on the planning of educational programs to move L.P.N.s to the A.D.N. level and A.D.N.s to the B.S.N. level has been significant— even though some educators might not be aware of the origin of the conceptual scheme that has initiated their curricular planning.

If we further refine the Wood model and interject the three-dimensionality of the interactive model for nursing practice proposed by the National Commission, we can develop an even finer description for each cube of that conceptual framework in terms of internal nursing levels, categories of specialization, and numbers of care providers needed to match expected client requirements. At the level of the statewide master planning committee, this model can be translated into how many A.D.N.s should be prepared for beginning practice competencies in distributive care settings rather than episodic environments, how many baccalaureate nurses should be prepared for primary care and how many for acute care, how many and what kinds of clinical specialists must be provided through graduate and/or certification programs, and how many nurses will be needed with advanced skills in research and inquiry.

In a democracy, there will always be a push and tug between planning and execution. Despite our best analyses of how many oncology nurses are needed with advanced clinical skills or how many clinical specialists are needed for burn units, freedom of choice or refusal is still a matter of fact. So long, however, as we visualize nursing as a mere aggregation or collection of individuals, without examining the differences in roles, levels, and environmental aspects of care, it is impossible to generate even the most simplistic kinds of projections that relate to the real world of health needs.

With a multidimensional concept of nursing, however, we can begin to describe the relevant characteristics of nursing roles in differentiated client care in such ways as to bring planning, preparation, and practice into a symmetrical and collaborative system. When that occurs, we will be able to speak meaningfully about nurse shortages and surpluses, retention and withdrawal, and, we hope, about career perspectives that will retain our best and our brightest in lengthy periods of full-time practice.

The vocational concept of nursing did not meet our needs for care. The occupational concept of nursing proved inadequate to the demands placed on it. The beginning professional model has suffered from an inability to differentiate levels and specialties—and the related preparatory routes—with the degree of finesse that is necessary for a complex system of health care. The emergent professionalization of nursing, with its multidimensional explication of nursing characteristics and concepts, is essential to the development of an adequate and properly poised body of nurse practitioners.

Having assembled evidence to indicate that the traditional concern over a nursing "shortage" is simply not well founded, we are left with the fact that our numbers have deceived us and that within our supply of nurses we have a surplus of some categories and a critical shortage of others. For the future, we must do a far better job of definition, of specification, and of targeting to ensure that we have sufficient numbers of nurses within each level and category of personnel. Only a multidimensional model will accomplish that goal.

EMERGENT TRENDS IN NURSING PRACTICE

Over the past decade, significant alterations in the form and organization of nursing practice have begun to unfold. Three of these deserve special attention as we look to the emergence of a full profession of nurse practitioners: primary nursing, the unification model, and the development of a parity model of organizational relationships. One or more of these concepts has been utilized in a variety of care settings, but perhaps the single institution that best exemplifies the combination of all three approaches in 1979 is Rush University of the Health Sciences together with its care component, the Rush–Presbyterian–St. Luke's health center. In discussing these developments, we shall draw primarily upon the Rush experience, particularly in terms of the interrelationships.

Primary Nursing Practice

In some aspects, primary nursing care is a throwback to the beginnings of nursing practice in this country, when much of a patient's treatment was given at home by private duty nurses who gave intensive individualized care around the clock. Beyond this point, however, the resemblance ceases because over the intervening decades, the knowledge base and the technology of physical and psychosocial nursing treatment have grown to the point where the historic pattern of private duty nursing would appear primitive by comparison. In human terms, however, there was a tremendous value in the nurse-patient relationship and in the clear recognition of individual responsibility for client care.

With the emergence of the hospital system in the United States in the early decades of the twentieth century, and with the reorganization of American medicine following the Flexner report, the locus of patient care and of nurse-patient relations shifted to the episodic treatment facility. The single nurse–single patient patterning of care gave way to the organization of wards and clinics in which groups of nurses provided care for groups of patients assembled usually in terms of maladies or injuries. The emphasis of nursing care was sharply focused on illness, the organization of nursing service became entwined with the medical care unit, and, most important, specialization emerged in terms of patient groupings. In order to care for large numbers of patients, functional nursing was adopted as a pattern for role configuration. Essentially, this was a task-oriented approach that developed not only out of the new technologies and demands for care, but also in relation to the broad effort in the 1920s to institute scientific principles of management throughout the organizations of our society. The division of work roles into clearly delineated tasks and job responsibilities matched neatly with the development of specific nursing duties that would somehow sum up into a complete coverage of patient needs. Hospital nurses increasingly found themselves performing a limited range of tasks —one might only take temperature, pulse, and respiration, for example, whereas another only passed medications—while patients found themselves encountering more and more individuals throughout their hospital stay. With the development of vocational nurses, nurse aides, attendants, and technicians, it was entirely possible for 40 individuals to see a single patient in the course of a day. Task responsibility might be fixed, but overall responsibility for care became diffused and dispersed.

In order to restore focus and direction to patient care, *team nursing* was proposed as an alternative to functional nursing. Nurses, aides, and attendants were to be organized into care teams under the direction of a professional nurse who was expected to be an expert in the clinical treatment of the patients handled by the team. In actuality, team nursing largely became a redeployment of role functions created under the earlier model of patient care. Nursing care might be planned by professionals, but it was largely delivered through others, the less qualified members of the team. Moreover, team leaders, whether head nurses or supervisors, were also responsible for administrative and management functions, which sharply reduced their ability to provide direct patient care. A number of studies on nurse utilization indicated that team leaders spent 80 to 90 percent of their time on administrative and institutional tasks, with the limited remainder being devoted to direct patient care. Moreover, because team assignments could vary from day to day and because turnover tended to alter the composition of the team at a rapid rate, patients still tended to see a large number of individuals and to experience a discontinuity of care and clinical direction.

Primary nursing care has evolved as a studied effort to provide individual attention and a planned continuity of care for each patient. In this reconfiguration of the nursing role, each patient is assigned a primary nurse who is responsible for the total nursing process throughout the course of treatment. (It is essential to recognize that the conceptual model of primary nursing is applicable to both episodic and distributive care and to in-patient and community or home facilities.) The primary nurse is expected to assess the patient's physical and psychosocial condition, make a diagnosis of individual care needs, draw up a plan for nursing care, follow the regimen of care determined, and conduct a continuous evaluation of that care and its outcomes. In the total conduct of this plan, the primary nurse will be assisted by a "nurse associate" who assists in providing care according to the plan prescribed, but it is the primary nurse who has total responsibility for patient outcomes 24 hours a day, 7 days a week.

The primary nurse not only develops the plan for nursing care, but also acts as the direct provider of that care as much as possible. This activity includes not only the ministration of functional tasks such as pulse and temperature recording, but also the provision of intravenous therapy, oxygen, or other specialized aspects of care. Administrative functions related to institutional management are systematically divested in favor of an enlarged scope of direct care. Understandably, this approach to nursing role explication requires greater nursing skills and more diversified practitioner competency. As a consequence, the number and percentage of registered nurses inevitably increases in relationship to licensed practical nurses, whereas the number of aides and attendants is dramatically reduced. Early efforts to assess the quality of care indicate that hoped-for improvements have come about and the response of patients, physicians, and families has been most positive [7].

Perhaps the most important element in primary nursing is its philosophic reassertion of the basic thrust of the profession—the scientific delivery of care, humanely dispensed, in accordance with the individual needs of patients and clients. More recently, at Rush University, the concept of primary nursing has been expanded to include family care that will involve patients, their spouses, and significant others in the planning and provision of care. This development proceeds from the observed importance of teaching and care instruction as performed by the primary nurse. The reduction of apprehension, the development of confidence, and the emergence of the patient as a positive participant in his or her own care are so essential to the planning, execution, and evaluation of the nursing plan that patient participation becomes a major component of the primary practitioner role. In enlarging that understanding to include a husband, wife, or other family members, the primary nurse practitioner is able to involve them in vital contributions to the patient's progress.

In sum, the concept of primary nursing has increased the identification of the practitioner with the patient, the physician, the family, and other health care professionals. It has enlarged the scope of nursing care and the accountability therefor. And, through the analysis of recorded data on quality of care, it has demonstrated the enhancement of patient treatment and the significant reduction of errors either of omission or of commission. Most important, it has increased the perceived professionalism of the nurse practitioners themselves, who have daily behavioral evidence of their enlarged role performance.

The Unification Model of Staffing

Closely entwined with the development of primary nursing in the Rush model for nursing is the reassertion of the need to bring nursing research, education, and service back into a single conceptual framework. All faculty members have responsibility for patient care and teaching—and are expected to contribute to the development of new knowledge related to the improvement of client care. Moreover, both undergraduate and graduate nursing students are taught regularly in the wards and departments of the health center, in both episodic and distributive settings, in ways that involve the nursing staff in the instructional process as well.

Beginning academic appointments are at the level of practitioner-teacher, a title that emphasizes the responsibility for the role occupant to both instruct and provide excellence in care. Thus, the faculty member is required to become a role model as well as a preceptor. Faculty promotions are based on the twofold growth of the individual; at the department-head level, the nurse is expected to serve in the dual position of clinical chief of service and academic head of the instructional program.

It is significant to note that the interaction between the nurses with joint appointments and those in nursing service has tended to have far-reaching impact. Over 65 percent of the entire nursing complement currently are baccalaureate graduates or higher, and this percentage continues to climb. Activity in in-service and continuing education is burgeoning as nursing service personnel respond to the challenge to work with the undergraduate and graduate students and to the opportunity to practice in what is described as a *center of excellence.*

To reward these individuals for their accomplishments, a system of so-called horizontal salary increments was installed. This was designed to increase the salary and related benefits of nurses and retain them in practice. Demonstrated growth in knowledge, clinical skills, and patient intervention, as well as in leadership, were analyzed in terms of a conceptual grid and clustered into a series of *zones of worth.* These, in turn, were designated as economic justification points for salary increases. As a result, there have been exponential improvements in patient care accompanied by increased nurse satisfaction [8].

The demands of the unification model are great, and there was a high initial rate of turnover at Rush among both the nursing service people, who were comfortable with the traditional arrangement of roles and function, and the practitioner-teachers, who found themselves unprepared to cope with the multiple elements of their positions. For the most part, these individuals were recent graduates of clinical master's programs and had had little or no preparation in pedagogy. With time, these problems were overcome. Turnover among nursing service personnel has declined, whereas the proportion of registered nurses (and registered nurses with baccalaureate or higher degrees) has climbed steadily. By providing in-service training opportunities in instructional planning, teaching, and evaluation, the more experienced faculty members have raised both the confidence and the accomplishments of their colleagues, and turnover among the practitioner-teachers has dropped significantly.

Nevertheless, personal on-site interviews underscore the fact that the unification role is still very challenging and that only individuals with ability and commitment can withstand the pressures induced by expectations held for the practitioner-teacher. Still, these pressures are to be expected in a consulting profession, and the Rush faculty are demonstrating that they can cope with the same demands that physicians and others endure daily in the same kinds of settings.

In the last analysis, the greatest impact of the unification model will come in the succeeding generations of students, who will be socialized in a setting where patient care and instruction are seen as companion elements in the performance of the professional role, where there is no false dichotomy between education and service, and where the nurse faculty member is a role model of clinical excellence to be imitated and admired. Only in this way can nursing emerge as a full profession, and the test of the unification model will lie in the willingness of its graduates to assume the burdens of practicing and teaching in the years to come, in whatever facilities or institutions they find themselves.

Reorganization for Parity in Roles

Implicit in the redesign of individual nursing roles for primary nursing and the unification model is the adjustment of the institutional organization to unleash the professional potential of this profession from the ceiling effect that traditionally has bound it in. Christman has argued that there must be a balance among the three major departments of medicine, nursing, and health administration but that this can be accomplished only through the development of an autonomous nursing staff that is explicitly permitted:

    1   The expression of clinical self-direction among nurses;
    2   The fulfillment of their responsibility to patients; and
    3   The acceptance of after-the-event sanctions rather than before-the-event controls over their practice [9].

Christman has developed an organizational framework for an autonomous nursing staff that can be operational in either a medical center or a nonteaching care facility. In the former situation, Figure 3–13, the deans of both medicine and nursing are also in charge of the administration of care throughout their service components. The deans relate to their respective staffs, which are arranged in congruent fashion for interprofessional cooperation in the planning and execution of patient care. Both the medical and nursing staffs have direct access to the governing board as well as to the deans so that they may present recommendations on policy and professional concerns. Implicit in this model is the recognition that nurses, like physicians, will be playing a full professional role in teaching, executing care, and pursuing the search for new knowledge to guide their praxis.

Each medical service unit has a related nursing service unit organized under a nursing chief who also has responsibility for the teaching conducted by the practitioner-teachers. Joint practice is reflected in joint decision making and in joint responsibility to the governing board for the excellence of patient care together with an economic use of capital and human resources.

Within the nonteaching care facility—whether it be a hospital, a health maintenance organization, or a large long-term care facility—a related but simpler organizational framework can be portrayed (see Figure 3-14). Composed of medical and nursing staffs and the administration, there would be the same equality and parity of role planning and functioning and the same access and responsibility to the governing board of trustees. In this case, since education would be of the in-service and continuing professional varieties, there would be no equivalent of the academic deanship. The heads of staff for both medicine and nursing would be charged with

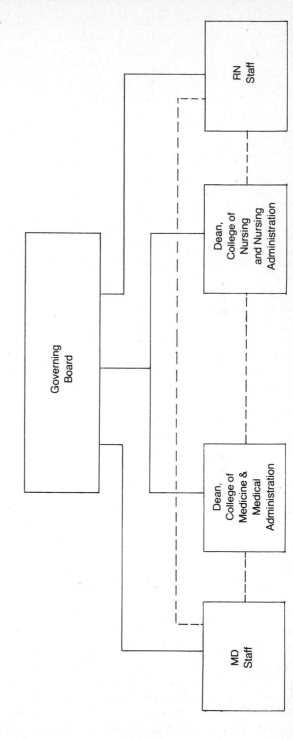

Figure 3–13 Schema for medical center hospitals. *(From Luther A. Christman, "The Autonomous Nursing Staff in the Hospital," paper presented under the auspices of the National Joint Practice Commission, June 9, 1976. Used with permission.)*

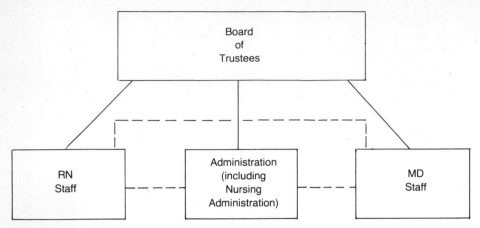

Figure 3–14 Schema for nonteaching hospitals. *(From Luther A. Christman, "The Autonomous Nursing Staff in the Hospital," paper presented under the auspices of the National Joint Practice Commission, June 9, 1976. Used with permission.)*

responsibility for providing training opportunities as needed and for encouraging their staffs to continue to update their knowledge and skill levels.

The concept of an autonomous nursing staff working in parity with a medical staff and with the central administration of the facility is the final explication of the full emergence of an unambiguous profession of nursing. It places full responsibility for the conduct of clinical nursing in the hands of nurses themselves and demands, in return, that nurses assume authority and accountability for the fulfillment of those role expectations. Medicine and administration rightfully should expect that nursing will assume total control of nursing care around the clock and through the year. Joint decisions do not absolve either clinical service from the responsibility to execute its functions with effectiveness, efficiency, and human concern. Joint policy making, joint planning, and joint practice admit of no scapegoating, and they allow for no timidity. Reliance on routines and regulations must give way to decision making, risk taking, and personal as well as professional reliability.

In short, an autonomous nursing service represents the clearest break with the traditional organization of nursing as a subprofession—acting on the one hand as an aid to the physician and on the other as an employee of the hospital administrator. At the same time, the autonomous nursing service is the best—perhaps only—way for nursing to document its unique contributions to health care delivery and patient benefits. The challenge is awesome, but the rewards are worth the stakes.

Knowledge as a Basis for Action

Woven throughout the emergent full professional model of nursing is the recognition that primary nursing, the unification model, and an autonomous nursing service are only as potent as the corpus of knowledge that guides them. The recombination of nursing education and practice is only preliminary to the addition of the research ability and capacity needed to achieve the triune nature of a full consulting profession. The opportunity for inquiry and discovery that is inherent in the new conceptual framework has been summarized by the nursing faculty at the University of Rochester in these words:

> Teaching is vitalized by delivering care to people and by the spirit of scientific inquiry. Such inquiry is encouraged by experience in nursing practice and by the questions of students and practitioners. Nursing practice in turn benefits from the latest findings through scientific inquiry and from challenge to staff members to serve as models of high quality practice for students [10].

It is in this light that nursing can begin to achieve its full potential, when practitioners raise questions that investigators then attempt to answer so that faculty members can incorporate their findings into instruction at the cutting edge of knowledge. Since in the emergent model of nursing organization, these three operations are carried on simultaneously by the same people, the probability of asking the significant questions, developing proper research models, and ensuring the translation of the knowledge acquired into both care and teaching is maximized.

Indicative of the growing interest in this activity is the study by Christ to identify the research priorities of nurses working in the unified organizational models at Rush University and the University of Rochester. Using the practitioner-teachers, master clinicians, and chiefs of nursing service as information sources, this investigator has sought to describe the current universe of needed research in these organizational exponents of the unification model and then group them in such ways as to develop a taxonomy of inquiry. The final step is to develop a priority system that can guide other investigators into those areas that display the greatest need or greatest probability of return in terms of patient benefit [11].

Although this approach may seem inconsequential to some and limiting in its effects on academic freedom to others, the probable benefits far outweigh the shortcomings. As Lindeman has suggested:

> A priority statement could be employed to interpret the significance of certain programs of research as well as to indicate the scope of nursing, for benefit of funding agencies, legislatures, and the public. Such a delineation of priorities could encourage the generation of new knowledge not only for the sake of knowledge but because of the potential social and professional benefits to be associated with or derived from knowledge [12].

In the near future, we will be able to examine the classification and priorities for research obtained from the unification models of teaching and service and, it is hoped, project an ordered set of inquiries that can become the focal point of a growing corpus of knowledge benefiting patients and the nursing profession through an enlarged scope of practice.

In the last analysis, the combined effects of primary nursing, unified practice, and autonomous nursing organization can go a long way in forging the links that can bind nursing together as a full profession. The development of knowledge and skill together with a mandate for discretionary authority and responsibility can lead to professional units that can solve the perennial problems of commitment and educational patterning. From this configuration there surely will develop that recognition of social worth which only the public can bestow. And it is the public ultimately which must accept nursing as a full partner and a full profession in the fabric of our health care system. If nursing does its part, the rest will follow naturally. In this new organization of forces, nursing has perhaps not only its best but its last chance to enter the twenty-first century as an integral element in the American health care system.

REFERENCES

1 "Extending the Scope of Nursing Practice," *A Report of the Secretary's Committee to Study Extended Roles for Nurses,* U.S. Department of Health, Education, and Welfare, November 1971.
2 Patricia McCormack, "Shortage of Nurses a National Problem," *Democrat and Chronicle,* Rochester, N.Y., September 23, 1979, p. 19a.
3 Ibid.
4 *NJPC Bulletin,* vol. 4, no. 2, December 1978, pp. 10–12.
5 "Educational Preparation for Nurse Practitioners and Assistants to Nurses: A Position Paper," American Nurses' Association, New York, 1965.
6 Lucile S. Wood, "Career Models for Nurse Practitioners," University of California at Los Angeles, Division of Vocational Education, Report of USDE Grant 8-0627, March 1972.
7 Regina Pryma, "Primary Nursing," *The Magazine,* Rush–Presbyterian–St. Luke's Medical Center, Chicago, Spring 1978, pp. 3 ff.
8 Luther Christman, "A Micro-Analysis of the Nursing Division of One Medical Center," in J. P. Lysaught (ed.), *A Luther Christman Anthology,* Contemporary Publications, Wakefield, Mass., 1978, pp. 83–87. See also Diane D. Elliott, "Faculty Response to the Assumption of Multiple Roles Within the Unification System of Collegiate Nursing Education," unpublished dissertation proposal, Graduate School of Education and Human Development, Rochester, N.Y., November 1979.
9 Luther Christman, "The Autonomous Nursing Staff in the Hospital," in Lysaught, op. cit., pp. 71–74.
10 "Faculty Research Development Grant Application," The University of Rochester School of Nursing to the Public Health Service, U.S. Department of Health, Education, and Welfare, 1977.
11 Mary Ann Christ, "Research Priorities in a Nursing Unification Model," unpublished dissertation proposal, Graduate School of Education and Human Development, University of Rochester, Rochester, N.Y., October 1978.
12 Carol A. Lindeman, "Priorities in Clinical Nursing Research," *Nursing Research* **23**: 693(1975).

Implementation of the Recommendations for Nursing Roles and Functions

In the initial chapter of its volume *An Abstract for Action,* the National Commission for the Study of Nursing and Nursing Education (NCSNNE) specified the primary objective for its entire investigation in these words, "Simply put, it is this: How can we improve the delivery of health care to the American people, particularly through the analysis and improvement of nursing?" [1]. High among the challenges of improved delivery of care was the lack of congruency between the traditional patterns of nursing roles and the changing demands for care coupled with the dynamics of scientific and technologic advancement.

Many persons—some nurses, more from outside the profession—viewed nursing as a relatively static occupation. Stereotypes abounded, and many of these had little to do with cure or care. One nursing leader was pained to say that flower arranging was seen by some individuals as a critical nursing skill. Significant differences were evident among physicians, administrators, nurses, and patients in their assessment of priorities for registered nurses [2].

To overcome these problems of both attitude and behavior, the National Commission recommended a broad-scale attack on several fronts. These included the need, first and foremost, for research into the actual effects of nursing intervention and care. Although personal opinion and bias about the benefits of nursing care were to be found in all directions, there was almost nothing in the way of hard data or evidence to document the real outcomes of the nursing function. Second, there was an evident need to redesign or reorganize the role relationships between nursing and the other clinical health professions, most particularly that of medicine. Sometimes it seemed as if new nursing functions were determined by what physicians wished to divest in terms of patient care. Little planning, less articulated effort, went into decision making for role change. A third problem area was the historic tie between nursing and the hospital. No one would dispute the need for competent care to be provided for the critically and acutely ill. Nevertheless, changing demands and economics of health argued persuasively for the development of nurses capable of maintaining health, preventing illness, and caring for the long-term patient with only slight impairment. In the past, public health nursing was sometimes treated as an add-on feature to a preparatory program in hospital nursing; for the future, nonhospital nursing needed to enlarge its own spheres of practice and role development.

Two other large-scale problems impinged on the nursing role. The first of these was the need for leadership, present and potential, for nursing service staffs—in whatever institution or agency they existed. The second was an assessment that changing technology and systems for delivery would affect all of the health sciences, including nursing, in significant, but largely unassessed, ways.

Taken all together, these five issues represented formidable barriers to the emergence of an unambiguous profession. Some of the matters were largely internal to nursing; some, such as that of role articulation with medicine, could be approached only through interprofessional planning and cooperation. All the concerns demanded change and innovation on the part of individuals who had long been afflicted with a low public image in these very categories of behavior and competence. Still, the National Commission was convinced that the very future of health care delivery in the United States was dependent upon the reconception, expansion, and extension of the nursing contribution to patient and client care over the full range of human needs. Ten years could not bring us conclusive solutions, but they could afford us the time for significant reorganization and growth.

With this aim in mind, the National Commission proposed both short- and long-term activities intended to foster change and growth in nursing roles and functions. In the next several sections, we shall examine the evidence related to the implementation of those proposals.

RESEARCH INTO NURSING PRACTICE

The National Commission assumed as a first principle that excellence in nursing practice resulted in measurable benefits both in improved aspects of care and in reduced costs of delivery. Unfortunately, at the time of the original investigation this belief could be substantiated by only meager evidence. Worse still, because of the lack of research into nursing intervention and practice, there were almost no guides for the improvement of nursing care beyond idiosyncratic belief systems. This situation, of course, is not unique to nursing. Almost every applied science has had to fight for acceptance of the concept that rigorous research is, first, possible in its field and, then, necessary and beneficial. So-called pure sciences and academic disciplines have been slow to accept and support the applied sciences, a situation that has had a profound impact on the training of researchers and the formulation of planning for high-quality investigations.

Indeed, it is hard to realize that American medicine, in 1910, was suffering from severe deficits in both a knowledge base and research capabilities. Medical training was based, according to Flexner, on the didactic presentation of a set body of doctrines of very uneven value. In order to upgrade the knowledge level of the physician and the student, it was recommended that schools of medicine be attached to research universities and that both basic and applied aspects of science be studied to assure optimum quality in patient care [3]. Perhaps no greater argument for the benefits of research can be advanced than the record of American medicine over the period from 1910 to the present. Transplants, implants, virtual elimination of many diseases, and the rehabilitation of countless individuals who might, only a few years earlier, have been doomed to misery are milestones along the length of that journey from Flexner to today. Life expectancy has increased not only in length but also in fullness, and medical research deserves our gratitude and support.

American nursing, however, still presented an impoverished figure in 1970 in terms of research capacity and support. There were very few nurses, less than 500, who had earned doctoral degrees, the generally accepted level for developed research competence. Moreover, many of these individuals had been trained in programs for educational administration or teaching; there were almost no doctoral graduates in nursing specifically prepared for research into clinical practice or nursing intervention. Additionally, there was little public or private support for nursing education. Many foundations had never been approached with a proposal for nursing research; only a few had ever given money for such a purpose. Of those foundations most disposed to assist nursing in educational or service areas, many had general prohibitions against helping basic or applied research, feeling that this was neither their purpose nor a field of expertise. Aside from some limited funds in the field of public health nursing, the federal government allocated no funds for nursing research until 1956, and it must be recognized that these were largely in the form of traineeships and other aids to advanced graduate education that included research training: only a limited amount was provided in the form of research contracts and grants.

To make a beginning in the development of nursing research, the National Commission recommended a minimum of $3 million in federal spending for nursing research in 1970, with a "desired" figure of $4 million. This money would be separate from some $15 million to $18 million intended for advanced graduate training at the master's and doctoral levels. As indicated in Figure 4–1, there has been a general rise in levels of federal funding for research over the period from 1968 to 1978, but it has been accompanied by sharp accelerations and declines from one year to the next; the figure for 1978 reached the highest point—just short of $6 million.

Overall, there is real satisfaction to be had in the doubling of the federal investment in nursing research over this decade. This pleasure must be tempered by the sobering fact that the Nixon and Ford administrations sought to impound some of these funds or to seek congressional approval for recision of the appropriated amounts. The Carter administration also sought reduction in appropriations and,

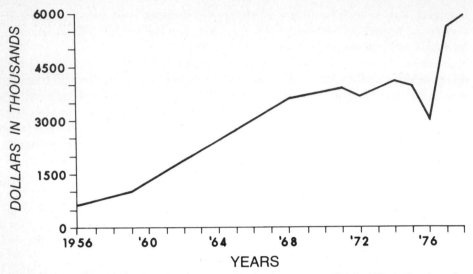

Figure 4–1 Federal funding for nursing research, 1956–1978. *(Original illustration based on figures supplied by the Division of Nursing, HEW.)*

more recently, vetoed the Nurse Training Act altogether. Some accommodation will surely be made, but the net effect has been to produce high levels of uncertainty and frustration in the situation. Researchers have found their projects approved with the proviso that actual funding must remain pending until some later point—time unknown—when the executive and legislative branches have agreed on specific amounts. Other researchers, in the midst of longer investigations, have learned that the continuation of their project is in a form of bureaucratic limbo awaiting a decision whether to operate on an emergency or interim budget until a compromise can be developed.

No one can be proud of the way these matters have been handled in recent years. It is easy to designate individual researchers and graduate students as the victims of the situation, but it is important to point out also that the general public is likewise affected. To the extent that greater knowledge of nursing interventions could lead to improved care and cost containment—as seems arguable from the record—then the populace as a whole is disadvantaged by the lack of support for nursing research.

The up-and-down character of federal financing has significance beyond its own final appropriations. Public agencies at the state or local levels tend to view federal activity in such an area as a confirmation or denial of need. Several states, for example, over the past decade have initiated or expanded programs for advanced nurse training involving research. Private foundations and corporations, too, have increased support for nursing research—often in programmatic areas of special interest, such as oncology, surgery, or neonatology. The overall picture is one of inadequacy, however, and the prospect for improvement requires a long-term view and commitment.

As an example of the current state of need, the American Nurses' Foundation

(ANF) was established to solicit and receive contributions and grants for nursing research. The largest portion of its income over the years, aside from a national start-up campaign, has come from the American Nurses' Association and the American Journal of Nursing Company. Less than 25 corporations and private foundations have made annual contributions to the ANF, and these have generally totaled less than $15,000 per annum, with the exception of certain designated funds for special projects. This low level of private outside support is reflected in the fact that only twice in the period from 1960 to 1976 did grants awarded by the ANF exceed the operating expenses—the fixed costs largely—of the organization [4]. In an effort to improve the effectiveness and efficiency of the operation and to seek increased involvement of the corporate and philanthropic sector in support of nursing research, the ANF was reorganized in 1978 and a board of directors was appointed entirely from the American Nurses' Association (ANA). There has been too little time at this point to assess the impact of the new leadership, but the need to develop greater resources to assist nursing research is obvious.

Another insight into both the needs of and the opportunities for nursing research comes from a survey of activities by the Southern Regional Education Board (SREB) [5]. Of a total of 207 identified research projects among educational institutions for nursing, only 59 (29 percent) reported funding for support of these efforts. Of that number, 40 (68 percent) were supported by the federal government, only 3 (5 percent) were supported by foundations, and 16 (27 percent) indicated some other form of aid, such as institutional funds or alumni support. Interestingly enough, of the 207 studies a majority (54 percent) were in nursing education and history whereas only 64 (31 percent) were in clinical subjects directly related to patient care. In contrast, there were 63 nursing research studies identified in the SREB area in federal agencies (military facilities, Veterans Administration hospitals, etc.). Of these, 55 (87 percent) related to nursing practice and only 2 (3 percent) related to nursing education.

Thus the continuation and expansion of funds for nursing research must be accompanied by a redirection of the purposes of that research, particularly among the institutions for nursing education. *The proper study for nurses is nursing,* and that must take precedence over other interests and issues. Research support should be expanded, but it should be better focused. There has been encouraging movement in this direction. The Commission on Nursing Research established by the American Nurses' Association has not only supported the better training of researchers and argued effectively for their support, but has also popularized the inclusion of research findings and reports in all professional meetings of the ANA. Likewise, the almost spectacular growth of the specialty practice groups in nursing has served as an energizer to both conducting and reporting of research. Research symposia and investigations at the cutting edge of clinical practice are common in the programming of meetings for the American Association of Critical-Care Nurses, the Nurses' Association of the American College of Obstetricians and Gynecologists, and many other clinical groups. These kinds of activities have generally encouraged support from pharmaceutical companies and other health-related corporations. The result is limited but growing contributions to clinical nursing research.

A monumental effort to reassert the centrality of clinical research to the professional development of nursing and, at the same time, establish priorities of need and importance is found in the investigative work of Lindeman [6]. Using the Delphi survey technique and a panel consisting of 419 nurses and 14 nonnurses, four rounds of weighted opinion seeking resulted in the identificaiton of clinical research needs and in the ranking of priority areas such as control of stress, treatment of pain, care of the aged, etc. The tabular rankings provide an unusually lucid guide for both researchers and funding agencies to utilize in developing and reviewing proposals for study. Lest there be a temptation toward a monolithic approach without consideration of unique needs, a lengthy minority report argues for the inclusion of other research concerns in a forceful way. The result is a document that argues for a set of widely perceived general needs, together with a broad distribution of alternative, or perhaps secondary, concerns. Already there have been two attempts to use this technique to develop more specific priorities within limited areas of clinical practice. Oberst, for example, has sought to establish priorities for cancer nursing research [7]; Christ is now completing an analysis of research priorities within a unification model for nursing practice [8]. Through such processes, greater refinement and clarity of purpose can be established for the specialized areas of clinical concentration.

One of the findings that emerged from the Lindeman study was a strong recognition that better dissemination was needed about research studies and their implications for nursing practice and that there was a related need to infuse learnings from research into both the educational programs and the treatment settings. This finding underscored a great concern found by the Commission in its initial study of nursing—that whatever the need for additional research in nursing, there was evidence that documented findings were not having the impact they deserved on teaching or practice. It was this shortcoming that prompted the Commission to recommend the establishment of a national clearinghouse for nursing research, to be placed presumably in the American Nurses' Foundation and supported by federal funds in the manner of the Educational Research Information Centers (ERIC) that were then being established across the country. This office would collect, abstract, and disseminate information on research and innovative developments in nursing and would develop the search and access systems that would allow inquiry from nurse teachers and practitioners on the state of the art of knowledge in their field at any given time.

It is one of the enduring disappointments of the Commission that the efforts to establish such a clearinghouse have been singularly unsuccessful. The Council of Nurse Researchers strongly recommended the establishment of a clearinghouse and information retrieval center, and this stand was supported by the Commission on Nursing Research of the ANA. Moreover, a proposal was developed by the American Nurses' Foundation to establish such a service and submitted to the federal Division of Nursing. The proposal was not approved for funding and apparently was not taken to any other federal agency for consideration under the guidelines of the ERIC program or the Library of Medicine. In personal interviews with staff members of the Division of Nursing in 1978 as a part of this longitudinal inquiry, it was indicated that the function could be handled by an extension of the Medlars system through the National Library of Medicine and that there was no need for a separate nursing clearinghouse. Shortly thereafter, an interview with the ANF staff indicated that the foundation had not shown any recent interest in establishing the type of clearinghouse described in the Commission's recommendation and had sought no funding for that purpose. More recently, however, the executive director of the ANF reported that the proposal has been revived and that the whole idea is under fresh examination.

There still seems to be a significant need to transfer nursing research findings to the clinic and the classroom. In the opinion of the Commission in 1970, the overwhelming amount of medical research in comparison with that of nursing argued against the inclusion of the latter in an extension of the health information retrieval systems. Moreover, some of the ERIC centers, with their expanded use of abstracting, annotation, and subject coding, represented attractive alternatives to some of the medical models. The growth in conduct and publication of nursing research argues for a proximate reconsideration of the issues and the options available, to ensure the broad dissemination and utilization of findings. There is no reason that a moderate fee for service should not be incorporated into the plan to provide continuing support; the basic question is whether nursing sees a need for a distinct system, or any system, for research dissemination and, if so, how best to get start-up funds to launch such a clearinghouse service.

In sum, there has been a dramatic increase in federal funding for nursing research which has generally been related to the recommended levels suggested by the National Commission. These funds, however, have often been used as pawns in political maneuvering, and the result is that planning and execution of research have often suffered through the vagaries of administrative and legislative battling. The general increase in federal funding over this period seems to have encouraged other public and private sources to assist graduate research training programs and support actual research grants and contracts. The need is greater than the resources, but the organized groups within nursing seem to have become much more sensitized to the need for and the benefits of research into practice and clinical intervention. The least progress has been made in the area of a clearinghouse or other device to facilitate the introduction of research findings into the teaching curriculum and the care setting. The momentum has quickened, but the distance to be traversed for nursing research to come of age is very great.

Perhaps, however, the near future may see some sort of breakthrough on multiple fronts of the research issue. Recently, the Division of Nursing funded a preliminary study for the development of protocols for the transfer of research findings into nursing practice at a faster rate. Jointly developed by the University of Michigan School of Nursing, the Michigan State University School of Nursing, and the Institute for Social Research, the project entitled the "Conduct and Utilization of Research in Nursing" (CURN) sought to identify and evaluate nursing research that is particularly suitable for transfer to practice settings. In retrieving, reviewing, and organizing studies into areas of conceptually related research, the project staff has developed a system that could well be the backbone of a complete clearinghouse for nursing research into client care [9].

Related to this CURN project is the effort mounted by Sigma Theta Tau, the recognition society for nurse researchers, to establish a clearinghouse through first organizing a registry of individuals and groups conducting research. This effort would be followed by the organization of a complete documentation and retrieval system much resembling the original concepts advanced by the National Commission. Funding must still be developed, but the efforts of the society may be the right approach to overcome the inertia that has set in since 1973 [10].

An encouraging sign of maturity in nursing research is also to be found in the emergence of new publications designed for researchers and for the consumers of their findings. In 1970, *Nursing Research* stood almost alone as a regular reporter of nursing research findings and generalizations. In 1979, we find nursing research included consistently in the specialty practice journals and in new periodicals devoted to the explication and transfer of research results. *The Western Journal of Nursing Research, Research in Nursing and Health,* and *Nursing Research Application Series* are indicative of nurses' new concerns for enlarging the corpus of their professional knowledge and transforming that increased understanding into the cutting edge of innovative practice.

Finally, the remarkable growth in the number of doctoral programs in nursing, a fourfold increase since the advent of the National Commission study began, gives promise of not only a greater supply of individuals trained for research, but also a definite commitment to the cardinal priority of such activities. In 1949, the first meeting of heads of graduate programs established the areas of administration, education, and supervision as targets for development. Today, the emergence of clinical master's programs that include concern for the utilization of research and the conduct of applied research has been complemented by the emergence of 20 doctoral programs in nursing, most of which are designed to develop investigative skills for conceptual and theoretical inquiry into nursing that will extend the scientific base of all nursing practice. That, in the end, will be the ultimate determiner of the professional status of nursing. There is much to be done, but the tools and the people are beginning to appear.

ROLE ARTICULATION IN HEALTH PRACTICE

Even before the publication of *An Abstract for Action,* it had become clear to a number of nurses and physicians that significant changes were taking place in the roles of both professions and that joint planning was necessary to fashion the most effective patterns for health care delivery. As indicated in Figure 4–2, nursing had largely begun to divest itself of the nonclinical assistive tasks that had once occupied a large portion of its daily work. Those activities that Christman has referred to as "stewardess" functions were gradually being reduced [11]. Simultaneously, nurses were moving into expanded clinical functions related to patient care both in areas associated with the nurse role and in fields that have long been viewed as the proper province of medicine. When nurses increased their ability to care for the psychosocial needs of patients, for example, this was simply a logical extension of their capacity as nurses. When those same nurses, however, were trained in physical assessment so that they could generate a primary diagnosis, then they were moving into an area long reserved to medical practitioners.

A series of national conferences on collaborative approaches to patient care were cosponsored by the American Medical Association (AMA) and the American Nurses' Association starting in 1964. Although these conferences were useful in many ways, it was obvious that a more systematic and detailed approach had to be taken to establishing new role relationships. It was obvious, too, that both professional groups would have to be open to change in order to develop matching and congruent roles. In 1970, the AMA Committee on Nursing approved the summary recommendations of the National Commission for the Study of Nursing and Nursing Education; subsequently, the trustees of the AMA endorsed the same recommendations at the urging of the committee, the latter group being then designated as the agency to work on specific activities related to the implementation of those proposals. From this beginning, steady and rapid progress ensued and, by 1971, the National Joint Practice Committee (NJPC) had been established by action of the AMA and ANA [12].

Over the 5 years that are the concern of this follow-up study, the accomplishments and contributions of the National Joint Practice Committee were substantial. In addition to continuing the holding of national conferences, the NJPC provided

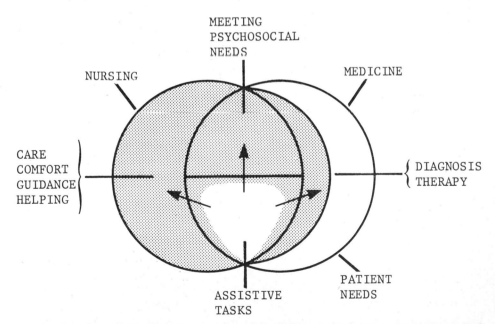

Figure 4–2 Trends in collaborative nurse-physician practice. *(From a conceptual framework of physician-nurse relationships developed by Barbara Bates, Robert Hoekelman, Harriet Kitzman, and Joan Lynaugh, all of the University of Rochester Schools of Medicine and Nursing.)*

ongoing and detailed analyses of the ways to effect improved patient care by altering roles of physicians and nurses. These were tested, documented, and reported in a volume entitled *Together: A Casebook of Joint Practices in Primary Care* [13]. A developmental study of four hospitals demonstrated the utility of joint practice in an episodic care institution. Among other elements, the project undertook to integrate patient records, develop joint patient care reviews, and enlarge the scope of clinical decision making by the nurses.

A number of significant statements were issued by the NJPC on matters relating to such interprofessional concerns as the certification of nurses and physicians and the passage of medical and nurse practice acts. These positions and recommendations not only served as guidelines for the professions themselves at the national and state level, but also were used by regulatory agencies, legislatures, and other professional groups as they examined ways to improve health care delivery. In particular areas, such as its study of the statutory regulation of the scope of nursing practice, the committee provided a wholly new resource for all those groups and agencies involved in registration and licensure. Finally, the NJPC provided extensive bibliographic and reference services to those interested in exploring the growing literature on joint nurse-physician practice in varied settings.

By any standard of measurement, the NJPC has been active in the pursuit of its aim to improve health care through the expansion of collaborative practice between nurses and physicians. In a series of interviews with the first four chairpersons, Genrose J. Alfano, Robert A. Hoekelman, Otto C. Page, and Shirley A. Smoyak, there was a considerable degree of consensus on the accomplishments and the disappointments over the years since the establishment of the Commission. All the interviewees agreed that substantial proof has been amassed on the effectiveness of joint practice and the complementary reorganization of both medical and nursing roles. There was a strong feeling that the discussions and negotiations that were required in order to plan and effect change were greater than anyone had anticipated —and that this interaction has to be a continuing process if the new professional relationships are to become truly effective. There was general agreement that the rank and file practitioners of both professions are still relatively unaffected by and uninvolved in true joint practice arrangements. In the opinion of these organizers of the NJPC, full realization of collaborative practice between nurses and physicians may be attained only when a new generation of both practitioner groups emerges from educational and training programs that are jointly organized and taught—that is, when student nurses and student physicians learn from their clinical beginnings to collaborate and cooperate.

One of the reasons that members of the NJPC may feel that they have not accomplished all they hoped for and the reason why so much emphasis was placed on statutory regulation is that, in our American system, we define and regulate both medical and nursing practice through 51 separate jurisdictions. This system can mean that procedures or interventions that would be permitted in Wyoming might be barred in New York and not even dealt with in Missouri. In turn, then, the only way in which the full scope of joint medical and nursing collaboration can be initiated is through action at the state level. Shortly after its organization, the Commission sought to encourage counterpart committees at the state level. As indicated in Table 4–1, there were 27 states that had joint practice committees in 1973. By 1978, this figure had increased to 41 based on a survey of the state nurses' associations. On the other hand, in 1973 there were only 3 states which had no vehicle for nurse-physician discussion of mutual problems, but this number had increased to 10 by 1978.

The significance of having joint practice committees at work in each state is underscored by the fact that 39 states indicated that there had been changes in their nursing practice acts since 1973, and another 6 were in the process of amending or enacting regulatory statutes. Of the remaining 6 states, at least half were contemplating the submission of proposed revisions. In all cases, the intent of the new or revised language was to enlarge the scope of professional nursing to "permit role evolution in accordance with the emerging features of health service." The fact that the NJPC had itself gone on record for more flexible and more broadly drawn statutes undoubtedly had some beneficial impact on the deliberations and actions that led to these positive conclusions.

It may well be that some of the feelings of disappointment over progress expressed by the leaders of the NJPC are simply the frustrations that most innovators experience over the slow pace of change. That this disappointment may be overdrawn is evident in the results of a 1977 survey of nursing service directors conducted by this study staff to determine, in part, the extent of "contagion" at the institutional level for the concept of joint practice committees. Although it is true that there have been collaborative committees of nurses and physicians for a long time, the concept of the joint practice committee to explore the role relationships of both professions can be dated to the enunciation of the National Commission's recommendations in *An Abstract for Action* in 1970. Using lists provided by the American Society for Nursing Service Administrators (ASNSA) and the ANA Council on Nursing Administration, a random sample of 392 institutions was drawn. Completed survey forms were received from 185 respondents, a return rate of 47 percent. In response to the question of whether the hospital had a "joint practice committee to plan and develop new, congruent roles for both nurses and physicians," it was surprising to us to learn that 87 of the respondents (47 percent)

Table 4–1 Number and Percentage of State Joint Practice Committees Established in the United States, 1971–1978

Year	Number of state joint practice committees	Percentage*
1971	0†	0
1973	27	53
1978	41	80

*The percentage is based on 51 jurisdictions: the 50 states and the District of Columbia.

†Several states in 1971 did have committees for liaison between the state medical society and the state nurses' association. These provided a precedent and help in establishing joint practice committees, but these earlier groups did not exist for the purpose of dealing with changed practitioner roles in both professions.

replied yes. Even more impressive was the fact that 75 percent of all university medical centers reported the existence of such committees while a majority of all community hospitals in the sample (54 percent) indicated an affirmative response. Teaching hospitals, Veterans Administration hospitals, and special-purpose institutions tended far less frequently to have organized bodies examining joint practice [14].

Among the institutions that did not have an overall joint practice committee, there were comments that certain specialty practice groups within the institution—particularly intensive care, the emergency department, and the delivery room—had departmental committees. Overall, 62 percent of these directors of nursing service reported that they saw evidence in their own institution of a "rearrangement of *both* medical and nursing roles in an effort to enhance patient care." Interestingly enough, most of the respondents felt that the joint practice concept had led to positive growth in professionalism of the nursing component as individual nurses became involved in more decision making related to patient care. Many respondents indicated that the involvement in joint practice had led to increased activity by nurses on peer review groups, audit committees, and medical staff committees at the department level.

When asked if, since 1973, there had been a change in the relationship between medicine and nursing, the nursing service directors, by a clear majority (63 percent), felt a significant increase in cooperation and harmony was in evidence. This improved professional relationship was most evident in the clinical unit, but was beginning to be seen throughout the organization. It must be added that a sensitive reading of the comments and appended notes would indicate that a millennium is not upon us and that there is a long way to go to achieve full collaboration. Many physicians still find it difficult to understand why nurses seek an expanded role—and many doubt whether nurses can function effectively in such a capacity. Many nurses are distrustful of physicians and see joint practice as simply a ploy to develop physician's assistants who will not truly share in decision making. Some nurses and some physicians simply feel no desire to change and experience discomfort even in its discussion. Perhaps this is why several directors of nursing service expressed interest in recruiting future staff from among students who had been exposed to joint practice in their educational preparation—a point earlier enunciated by several of the organizers of the NJPC in surveying the national scene.

In contrast to the view of the nursing service directors, our study staff also inquired of the state nurses' associations how they viewed acceptance of an expanded role for nursing in the provision of patient care. In their view, the greatest acceptance lay among patients, then among other nurses, and thirdly among nurse administrators. These groups were followed in descending order by physicians, nonnurse administrators, and third-party payers. It is essential that the objective viewer recognize that these somewhat disparate opinions actually convey reality. The closer the nurse and the physician find themselves together with the patient, then the better the likelihood of collaboration and cooperation. At the same time, the feelings of the professional organizations at national, state, and local levels become powerful influences on the pace and directions of change.

In terms of the next several years, it is vital for the developing health care system of this country that the NJPC, along with the AMA and ANA, continue to provide leadership and encouragement to the concepts of joint practice. The Commission and its parent bodies should provide assistance and support to the state counterpart committees and, in particular, continue to address the particular problems that have stood in the way of establishing joint practice committees in 10 states. If the testimony of the past 7 years is to be believed, then patient care would benefit from a concern for professional collaboration and nurses and physicians would find increased cooperation a constructive way to more rational relationships. It is hard to believe that no problems involving role expectations or overlap exist in the states that have no joint practice committee. The establishment of such a group is no cure-all, but it is a step toward recognizing and defining the real problems that do exist between these two professions—and the stake that the public has in the improvement of health care delivery.

To those original Commissioners and staff of the NJPC, our society owes much that few will truly comprehend. To their expressions of disappointment or shortcoming, perhaps the best reply is to paraphrase the words of Dr. Samuel Johnson: "If some readers find that something is omitted, let them also recognize that much has been accomplished." The vitality of the national body, the substantive growth of state counterpart committees, and the increasing evidence of collaboration on joint practice at the institutional level are an impressive record of accomplishment and dedication. The clear relationship that directors of nursing service and others see between joint practice and improved nurse-physician collaboration is an eloquent measure of success.

ORGANIZATION OF NURSING ROLES

As the National Commission viewed the roles and functions of American nursing in 1968, three closely related but distinct problems emerged. Taken not in order of importance but in terms of a conceptual schema, these were the lack of role differentiation among nurses, the lack of an expanded role expression for clinical expertise, and the separation of education from practice with resultant deprivations for both groups. In the following pages, each of these problems will be considered in light of the National Commission's recommendations to overcome these concerns and the evidence on progress toward implementation.

Role Differentiation in Nursing

Because the first training schools for nurses were organized in hospitals—and some of them by female physicians rather than nurses—it is quite logical that the curriculum for training should follow closely the pattern for medical service in an inpatient facility. Instructional courses, clinical experiences, and, indeed, licensure examinations reflected the medico-hospital quadrivium of medicine, surgery, obstetrics, and pediatrics. Psychiatric nursing was added much later and was regarded by some nurse educators as "fluff" introduced simply to assuage the collegiate students and their faculties who wanted some relief from the "hard" elements of the curriculum.

Early in its study of nursing, the National Commission became convinced that programs for nursing education—whether in hospital schools, associate-degree colleges, or baccalaureate institutions—represented specialized routes for education, training, and socialization into the acute care facility. To label the resultant curricula as general was at best a contradiction of terms.

At about the same time, the Citizens Commission on Graduate Medical Education argued that most medical care was a "repair service" and that significant changes had to be made in our approach to training and practice [15]. Estimates from a variety of sources suggested that as much as 88 percent of our health care problems simply had nothing to do with hospitalization or acute illness. The problems of keeping people well and of handling mild unwellness or illness, the maintenance of the chronically unwell—all these concerns affected many more people on a continuing basis. At the same time, these nonacute problems were held in low priority by many of the practitioners in medicine or nursing and involved the institution of the hospital even less.

The recognition of this phenomenon was not new. The original study of American nursing, the Goldmark Commission of 1923, had emphasized the need for public health nursing as a corollary to hospital nursing. Succeeding examinations into nursing confirmed the basic necessity of some new configuration in nursing practice and education. In the course of site visits and data collection in the late sixties, the National Commission confirmed by observation and data collection what so many others had arrived at by intuition and discussion: nursing practice had, indeed, anticipated the educational processes and curricula, and individual nurses were already practicing along a complex continuum of situations involving three variables. As indicated in Figure 4–3, there are a variety of behaviors in nursing based on patient need. These can generally be classified as assessment, intervention, and instruction. On another plane, the patient or client condition can be described as well, mildly unwell, or acutely unwell. On a third dimension, the environmental setting may vary from an institution to a short-term facility to a home or office setting. What our investigations concluded was that there was a description of almost factorial accuracy that could be used to delineate the exact combination of practice requirements in any combination of interventions, patient conditions, and environmental locations. In an effort to reduce complexity and to group the varieties of nursing practice under some general statements of condition, the staff devised the classifications of *episodic* and *distributive* care using these definitions:

1   Episodic care is that domain of nursing practice that is essentially curative and restorative, generally treating ill patients, and most frequently provided in the setting of the hospital or other in-patient facility;

2   Distributive care is that domain of nursing practice which is essentially designed for health maintenance and disease prevention, is generally continuous in nature, seldom acute, and increasingly will take place in community or emergent care settings.

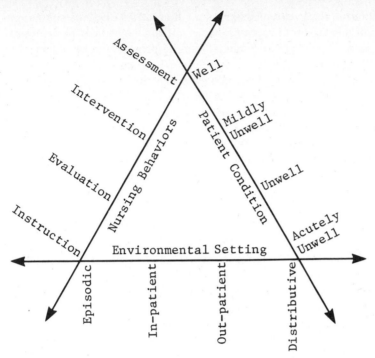

Figure 4–3   Interactive model of three variables in nursing practice.

Despite the fact that many nurse educators responded with concern bordering on hostility, the fact is that these general definitions matched the analyses of several other contemporary studies of nursing roles and functions. Esther Lucile Brown's thorough analysis of institutional and community nursing care; the Advisory Committee to the Secretary of Health, Education, and Welfare; and the World Health Organization Working Group used different terminology but assessed the same root need for differentiated nursing practice to meet a broad range of client care needs from an acute point to that of simple health maintenance.

The National Commission proposed that two distinct but related "concentrations"—episodic and distributive role performance—be developed for nursing education and practice with further specialization to be developed beyond the preparatory stage. In a series of surveys conducted by this study staff in 1977–1978, it was apparent that a positive response has begun to emerge. In a random sample, striated by the kinds of institutional governance of preparatory nursing programs, it was indicated that 37 percent of all responding schools of nursing had provided clinical concentrations in episodic or distributive care whereas another 29 percent had provided some form of differentiated clinical concentration using some other conceptual scheme or terminological definition. In toto almost three out of four of the responding institutions for preparatory nursing education have begun to move away from the traditional viewpoint that all nursing education is hospital nursing education and had begun to develop viable clinical alternatives at the introductory level. Within the differing kinds of programs, baccalaureate institutions have moved most rapidly (78 percent) whereas community college programs have shown the least elasticity (50 percent).

A survey of state nurses' associations indicates that the growing emphasis on differentiated practice in nursing was becoming evident to the professional organizations. Of the respondents, no less than 32 states (63 percent) reported that there was "pronounced" growth in distributive care practice within their state since 1973, and an additional 6 states (12 percent) reported that there was evidence of "some" growth in distributive care. The remaining 13 states (25 percent) saw no evidence of a fundamental shift in role concentrations and practice behaviors. Our inquiry directed to hospital directors of nursing service, even though they might be expected to be interested in nurses prepared for episodic practice, indicated that more than one out of four (27 percent) were looking for differentiated clinical skills within the general domain of episodic care.

In one sense, the National Commission had little investment in the specific terms *episodic* and *distributive*. They were intended to provoke thought and to get people away from such stereotypic labels as *hospital care* and *public health nursing*; in large part, we thought those designators were hackneyed and unidimensional. If the terms of the Commission caused ferment, they also caused reexamination of both education and practice. In less than a decade, more than a third of our sample institutions identified with this terminology but, more important, with its underlying concepts of diversity and choice. A smaller but almost equal number of institutions were providing choice under another rubric or schema. Taken together, these figures indicated that education was catching up rapidly on the practice roles and functions that prompted the recommendations for differentiated concentrations in clinical preparation and intervention, and this progress was further underscored by the evidence that the institutions and settings for health care delivery were following suit by providing room and scope for practitioner diversity.*

The growth of primary nursing, the innovation of health maintenance organizations, and newer forms of health insurance have helped in the initiation of change. By current projections, these forces should continue and validate the need for greater differentiation in nursing practice based on a complex, rather than simplistic, analysis of client needs and nursing behaviors. If the principle is not triumphant, it seems to be well established and quite durable.

Expanded Clinical Roles

To those from outside the field of nursing, one of the most surprising of the National Commission's findings was that the greater the length of experience of nurses in the hospital setting, the less involvement they were likely to have in direct patient care. Promotion patterns and increased compensation essentially took nurses more and

---

*Indeed, in our site interviews, some observers mentioned concern that colleges and universities were moving too rapidly away from episodic curricula and felt more emphasis should be placed on preparation for care of the critically ill.

more into management of things and away from the care of people. The reasons were plain enough, but unacceptable from the standpoint of enhancing the delivery of care. In the evolution of the American hospital system, there was almost no professional preparation of administrators until after the Second World War and, consequently, almost no developmental route for the training of middle management levels. Because nurses represented the most plentiful supply of capable personnel available, they were drafted into the supervision and management, not of nursing, but of the hospital as a business enterprise. A host of studies confirmed that nurses at the first level of promotion—as head or charge nurses—spent less than 20 percent of their time in direct patient care, and supervisory nurses, those at the second level of promotion, spent much less than 10 percent of their time in care activities.

There was a second reason, as well, for the inverse relationship between nurse experience and patient involvement. All too often, there was a virtual ceiling effect placed upon the role of the nurse. Although many people spoke openly to our study staff in the sixties about how nurses performed all kinds of tasks—especially from 3 in the afternoon to 7 the following morning—there was an aura surrounding these activities that bordered on illegitimacy. Nurses delivered babies—but only under extreme circumstances. Nurses prescribed and administered medications—but only when the physician could not be reached. Nurses wrote orders—but they were signed or countersigned by the doctor the next day. To the insider, this was the way things were and had been. To the outsider, this was an almost conspiratorial approach to expanded nursing roles.

On closer examination, the answer, in the opinion of the National Commission, lay somewhere in between. Nursing education, from its inception, had been so occupied with preparatory programs that little had been done in the area of advanced clinical training. Those programs that existed for the postpreparatory education of nurses were largely in education or administration—almost none were in clinical practice. Thus, a nurse in an expanded role was, almost by definition, an experienced individual who had developed a personal bond of trust and confidence with one or more physicians such that this nurse became an exception to the rule. This highly idiosyncratic situation meant that any change in the personal equation might reduce the function of the nurse to a base level. If the nurse or the physician moved to another institution, it often meant the slow and careful rebuilding of clinical, professional, and personal relationships.

Beginning in the midsixties, however, a marked change began to take place in graduate nursing education. A large number of clinical master's programs were established, and their enrollments flourished. In the decade beginning in 1968, the total number of master's degree enrollments more than doubled, from 3000 to 6000, and the percentage of clinical students rose from one-third to three-fourths. The percentage of enrollment in teaching fell from 44 to 16; the percentage of enrollment in administration fell from 10 to 5; the percentage of enrollment in supervision fell from 12 to less than 1. Over this same period of time, more and more physicians sought help in meeting the strident demands for increased delivery of health care by supporting specialized programs in a variety of fields to produce *nurse practitioners*— individuals with advanced diagnostic and therapeutic skills.

These changing patterns in nursing and medicine converged to produce, for the first time, a significant number of nurses who were prepared formally to practice in an expanded role. In projecting the impact of this development, the National Commission proposed that medicine, nursing, and health administrators adopt a three-level conceptual scheme for the legitimation and expansion of the clinical nursing role in a rational and planned manner. As indicated in Figure 4–4, each professional nurse would be expected to function effectively in a scientific approach to patient care, that is, every nurse would be involved in patient assessment, diagnosis, care planning, care provision, and the evaluation of outcomes. The chief distinction at the staff nurse level would be the effort to think and practice in terms of conceptual wholes and scientific relationships, rather than on the basis of discrete procedures or interventions.

Above the staff nurse level, the distinctions between the proposed system and the traditional arrangement of nursing service would become even more acute. Head nurses, charge nurses, supervisory nurses, and assistant directors—all with their emphases on nonpatient tasks—would be swept away, their duties to be taken up by properly prepared middle-level health administrators. The second-level nurse practitioner, termed the *clinical nurse* in the NCSNNE design, is a leader in clinical care with an expanded armamentarium of cognitive, affective, and psychomotor skills in the full range of scientific care planning and execution. The third-level nurse practitioner, the *master clinician,* would serve as the organizer of complex care and the role model for first- and second-level practitioners.

By 1973, the National Commission in *From Abstract into Action* could cite a number of case examples of planned role expansion in both episodic and distributive care settings which established the basic soundness of the proposal [16]. Much more experimentation and development was needed, however, to prove that large numbers of nurses would accept the increased responsibility of an expanded practice and that their activities could be fashioned into a congruent pattern of physician-nurse collaboration. In terms of this longitudinal study, then, we were looking for evidence

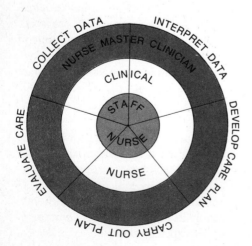

Figure 4–4 Three-level conceptual scheme for the development and expansion of nursing practice.

of expanded clinical roles for nursing which displayed developmental stages, objective benchmarks for distinguishing those stages, and a formulated approach to professional growth along the stages.

Although the recommendation for the trilevel formulations of the National Commission enunciated in 1970 was based, in large part, on the observation of some nurses in advanced clinical practice, much of it had to be conjectural and projective because there were no demonstration programs that could be examined and evaluated. Over the intervening years, however, additional experience refined the concept of expanded nursing roles. The Nurses Association of the American College of Obstetricians and Gynecologists (NAACOG), in April of 1979, provided an amended definition of nursing titles based on its clinical requirements and the insight gained through the effort to document and certify significant differences in levels of care provision [17]. The association saw a three-level system also, but with a differentiation within the second level of practice. The approach to the expanded role was as follows:

Level 1 *Professional Nurses.* Graduates from an accredited preparatory program licensed to practice. Able to provide direct care to patients utilizing the nursing process.
Level 2 *Nurse Clinicians.* Professional nurses who demonstrate expertise in nursing practice and ensure ongoing development through clinical experience and continuing education. This role is recognized by means of certification.
Nurse Practitioners. Professional nurses prepared in a specialized education program with emphasis on certain diagnostic and therapeutic knowledge. This role is recognized by means of certification.
Level 3 *Clinical Nurse Specialists.* Professional nurses with advanced knowledge and skill in a specialized field. Prepared at the master's level with an emphasis on specific areas of clinical nursing. This role is recognized by means of certification. Clinical nurse specialists provide direct care and plan and guide the work of others. Particularly they promote and utilize research in the improvement of care practices.

Certain liberties have been taken by this study staff in abridging and emphasizing elements of the NAACOG definitions, and we invite those interested to read the original documentation. The unique contribution of this scheme to the understanding of role staging and expansion in nursing, however, lies in the specification that the middle level of practice actually involves two compatible but distinct groups of experts: one, the nurse clinician, is still a generalist albeit a very competent practitioner; the second, the nurse practitioner, is becoming a specialist in terms of elements of the scientific nursing process. The NAACOG definition speaks of diagnostic and therapeutic knowledge, but one might also emphasize evaluation or other areas of scientific care as viable alternative areas of specialization. At the third level, the clinical nurse specialist, the generalist and specialist essentially combine through a combination of advanced training and practitioner experience.

In an effort to assess the actual impact of the expanded role in care institutions, we queried our national sample of nursing service directors on their analysis of several specific elements of the concept. For example, any expansion of the nursing role should affect the ratio of clinical functions to those of institutional maintenance. We asked the directors of nursing service whether there had or had not been a significant increase in the proportion of time devoted to direct patient care by their nurses. Seventy-one percent of the respondents replied yes. Twenty-two percent found no real change. Again, the conceptual scheme advanced for the expansion of the practice role would argue that promotions should be based on clinical expertise rather than on administrative capability. Seventy-three percent of the directors of nursing service say that their institutions expect and in fact require that supervisory nurses be more clinically competent than the staff nurses they direct. Interestingly enough, however, only 61 percent of the hospitals surveyed based their reward and recognition systems solely on clinical competence.

This somewhat paradoxical situation is attributed to the growth of bargaining unit contracts, wherein seniority must be considered as a prime factor in advancement, and the need to retain older service individuals even in a noncontractual system where an acute local shortage of nurses is a common phenomenon.

More to the point, however, in terms of actually implementing a system for advanced clinical roles is the reorganization of nursing service to provide positions and budgetary support for differentiated levels. Here the results are not so encouraging. Only 27 percent of the responding institutions, for example, had actually hired nurse practitioners to carry out the defined competencies of the second level, although the differentiation on this point was marked among the kinds of hospitals concerned. Eighty percent of the Veterans Administration hospitals reported hiring nurse practitioners; at the other extreme, community hospitals indicated that practitioners were employed in only 18 percent of the sample surveyed.

If there is any consolation in this situation, it may be in the fact that 36 percent of all the reporting institutions had already designated certain clinical positions in nursing to be filled only by a certified practitioner with advanced clinical skills. Budgetary restraints, lack of available applicants, and bargaining contracts were again cited as problems. Some public institutions added the fact that job classifications and occupational coding required drastic updating before advanced-level practitioners could be appointed or paid competitive salaries.

On the basis of these surveys, site visits, and interviews, an objective statement of the situation on expanded clinical roles might be this: There is general agreement among nurses, physicians, and administrators that these concepts are here to stay and will grow; at the time of the survey, most facilities and agencies have a truncated approach to levels of expanded nurse role; about one out of every four hospitals have some form of approach, but among these, some have only the first two levels, some have adopted a first-and-third-level combination that ignores the middle-level-practitioner concept; and perhaps as few as 30 or 40 institutions in the whole country have moved to a graduated three-level plan for the expansion and reformulation of nursing practice. One indication that the road may be turning, however, is the fact that, among the heads of nursing education programs, the issue of expanded roles is seen—far and away—as the most significant trend of the 5-year period. Practice precedes education, but practice must then wait for education to provide the "critical mass" of trained people who can carry innovation into the realm of universal implementation.

Two developments in care facility staffing patterns suggest that movement toward better professional utilization is under way on a large-scale basis. Primary nursing, the concept of having a designated nurse responsible for all phases of patient care for a specified case load of clients, is being experimented with—or adopted— by a number of hospitals, long-term facilities, and health maintenance organizations. Undoubtedly, the prospects are for greater application of this approach in the near future. Relatedly, the movement toward a staff of all registered nurses is gaining momentum, particularly in hospitals, as a way to ensure greater quality of care while reducing the overall numbers of individuals involved in providing that patient care.

High on the list of priorities for making nursing into an unambiguous profession must be the emergence of a clear career pattern based not on subsidiary elements, but rather on the primary focus of clinical excellence. The emergence of expanded levels of competency, the documentation of differences that really matter, and the recognition and reward of those behaviors are essential to keep the "brightest and the best" in nursing. To date, a start has been made but the emphasis on practice and the pursuit of clinical commitment is still not sufficiently affirmed. If the study of nurses is nursing, so too, then, the business of nurses is nursing. No one can do it better; no one can do it as well. It is nurses who will determine the final extent of competency and excellence.

Unification of Education and Practice

In the early strivings for the establishment of a collegiate system for nursing education, there was a healthy unhappiness with the relationship between the hospital and the diploma school of nursing. Early studies of the profession emphasized the lack of educational quality, the preeminence of concern for staffing needs over teaching, and the outright exploitation of students in many institutions for the benefit of the parent organization.

When separation occurred, it came with a completeness that contained many unanticipated consequences. Collegiate nursing faculty often found themselves in academic institutions that had no clinical components; indeed, in some cases there was a considerable physical separation from the nearest care facility. Nurse faculty interacted with colleagues who had little comprehension of the actual demands for preceptorial teaching and had little sympathy for what they saw as unusual student-faculty ratios or time away from the classroom setting. Moreover, the standard practices for promotion and tenure in the collegiate institution typically centered on scholarly research and publication rather than practitioner expertise in a clinical field.

On the other hand, the nursing service people in hospitals found that the accelerated demise of the diploma programs tended to isolate them just as effectively from nursing education. Communications deteriorated, and when nurse educators arrived with students, nursing staffs complained that the students were taught only "ivory tower theories" or, alternatively, that the responsibility for clinical instruction was "dumped" on nursing service because the school people were not up to date in practice.

Granted that these points are sketched out with hyperbole. Nevertheless, the fact is that nursing educaton and service drew apart in ways that were detrimental to each other and most harmful to the student. Unlike the "full" professions of medicine and dentistry, whose faculty continued their identification as practitioners, nurse educators and service personnel frequently worked in splendid isolation—even to the extent that some diploma school faculty were seen as too removed from the care concerns of their own institution and incapable of practicing what they taught with any degree of excellence.

As the National Commission pondered the data from interviews and surveys on the troubled relationships between education and service, between teaching and practice, it seemed that, ultimately, nursing must elaborate a unified model for professional socialization and practice—a professional community of *nursing*. The details of the curriculum and the behaviors associated with care should be that of nursing, but the general formulation of the model should place ultimate responsibility for both teaching and role modeling on the clinical faculty. As in medicine, we should expect to see practitioners teaching students, at both preparatory and advanced levels, in the classroom or clinical unit, and then demonstrating their continuing ability to care for patients on a regular, protracted basis with evidence of effective outcomes.

Parenthetically it should be added that most of the new advanced clinical programs, either for nurse practitioners or for master's degree students, found their first requirement lay in updating and "refreshing" the skills of nurse faculty so that they could exhibit the assessment, care planning, and intervention that they were required to display.

As short-term approaches to the reunification of nursing education and service, the National Commission proposed that interinstitutional cooperation be broadened and that joint appointments and personnel utilization be fostered in both directions, that is, to encourage outstanding practitioners to engage in teaching activities and to facilitate the adoption of patient care responsibilities by faculty members. In 1977 and 1978, we sought to determine from directors of nursing service and education just how far these developments had gone. The directors of nursing service indicated that only 28 percent of their hospitals had officially appointed nurse educators to positions in nursing service directly related to patient care. Seventy-five percent of the university hospitals and 100 percent of the Veterans Administration hospitals, however, had taken this action, and community hospitals, the most numerous subset, registered 28 percent activity. Asked if they provided joint appointments of their nursing staff to the faculty of educational institutions, 27 percent of the respondents replied affirmatively. Again, university and Veterans Administration hospitals led the way in these activities, with community and special-purpose hospitals participating least.

Perhaps a little more interpretation of these findings is provided by the survey results from the educational institutions. When asked if their institution encouraged appointments that included responsibility for client care *and* teaching, only 40 percent of the institutions replied affirmatively, but 61 percent of the baccalaureate institutions sampled indicated that this type of appointment was encouraged. Relatedly, only 32 percent of all the educational institutions provided academic appointments for nursing service personnel, but 65 percent of the baccalaureate institutions did so.

In effect, then, baccalaureate institutions, university hospitals, and Veterans Administration hospitals seem to be at the cutting edge of increased interaction and joint appointments. Hospital schools of nursing, associate degree programs, community hospitals, and special-care facilities have moved the least in these directions. Among the reasons cited for failure to become involved in these arrangements were budgetary restrictions, geographic isolation, difficulties of time sharing on a continuing basis, and the lack of appropriate credentials for formal appointment to another institution. These are real problems, but it is significant that many educational programs and care facilities have surmounted the same difficulties. At least some of the inaction lies in inertia—some of it in old biases and prejudices that are still far from overcome. The problem may also lie in the fact that some nurse faculty members simply cannot or will not become involved with patients.

In a small but growing number of institutions, the gradualism of joint appointments and enlarged cooperation has been waived in favor of a bold new approach to a "unification" model of nursing service and education. Perhaps the first studied effort to restore partnerhood between teaching and practice on a scientific and conceptual basis—as well as at the pragmatic level—was the experiment at Case–Western Reserve [18]. Faculty and nursing service personnel worked to expand the role of nursing practice and to enhance care and teaching through heightened interaction and joint planning. The difficulties of doing this in even one hospital service were far greater than anticipated, but the outcomes were most promising [19].

By 1972, following the continued experimentation on smaller adaptations of the unification model and with the steady growth of clinical master's programs that provided a new resource for academic appointments, two large-scale organizational innovations were initiated. The Rush University of the Health Sciences and the University of Rochester launched programs designed to pull nursing service and education together into a single framework that would, moreover, establish parity as nearly as possible with all other clinical departments of their institutions—but most particularly that of medicine [20, 21].

The dean of the school of nursing would also be director of nursing service. Below the office of the dean would be departments that would undertake the full professional scope of practice, teaching, consultation, and research. Each department would be headed by a qualified nurse, optimally prepared at the doctoral level, who would serve as the clinical chief for that nursing service and as the academic department head. The middle-level role in nursing care would be undertaken by practitioner-teachers, graduates of master's programs in clinical care, or nurse practitioners prepared in specialized clinical programs. The first-level practitioners would be graduate nurses, licensed to practice, involved with both students and patients.

The implications of these organizational arrangements are far-reaching in terms of a full profession of nursing. For the first time, schools of nursing have subscribed to the proposition that they will carry full responsibility and authority for operating as an equal partner of their colleagues in medicine. (Christman, at Rush, uses the term *parity* in preference to *equality* to connote the fact that there are and should be differences in specific arrangements based on real distinctions in treatment modalities, care objectives, practitioner skills, and collaborative planning.) Appointments to the school of nursing are made in the expectation of contributions to care and to teaching. Promotion and tenure are to be based on the combined assessment of clinical excellence, teaching performance, and scholarly activities.

By emphasizing the need for doctoral graduates at the third level of the nursing role and that for master's graduates at the second level, both Rochester and Rush are moving as far as the present limits of the profession will allow. There are simply not enough doctorally prepared nurses available to provide, for example, full equality with medicine in terms of academic preparation, person for person, rank for rank. But these approximations materially reduce the educational and clinical gap that has long existed between medical and nursing staffs in most care settings. Moreover, the assumption by the unified nursing body of responsibility for everything that takes place in the name of that profession increases accountability and reduces scapegoating between separate entities for care and teaching.

Visits and interviews with nurse practitioner–teachers at these institutions confirm the increased pressures that come from the unification model. The more traditional the individual—either faculty member or nursing service member—the more difficult it is to carry out the combined role. At the same time, for many nurses there is a tremendous exhilaration in the challenge to make nursing a full citizen in the clinical academic community. And, over time, the feeling of accomplishment increases as challenges are met and as experience is gained in the new professional roles. Successive administrations of the Nursing School Environment Inventory to the Rush University practitioner-teachers over the period from 1975 through 1978, for example, revealed increases in general esteem, academic enthusiasm, intrinsic and extrinsic motivation, breadth of interest, and encapsulated training [22]. Over the same period of time, the rate of turnover throughout the nursing population was reduced and the rate of stability was sharply increased (an indication that much of the remaining turnover could be attributed to new arrivals who quickly sensed that the Rush system was not for them). Another example of the impact of the new organization is to be found in the overall configuration of the staff population of nursing over the 5-year period. In 1973, 64 percent of the staff were non-R.N.s; in 1978, despite an increase of 125 positions, the staff was composed of 71 percent R.N.s. This significant reversal in staffing patterns is a natural result of the expansion of the nursing role and the redefinition of levels of practice and knowledge required for the exhibition of the unification model of institutional organization [23].

Much remains to be done at Rush, at Rochester, and at an increasing number of institutions that are adopting or adapting these models to their own environmental requirements. In the whole evolution of nursing education, perhaps no other development will hold the significance of the remarriage of care and teaching in a major clinical facility, with its emphasis on research and scholarly activity firmly based on a clinical foundation. The problem with the original model of nursing education was that it often subverted education to service. The reaction often meant an overemphasis on didactics and a bare threshold level of clinical experience. The model of the future may well lie in the unification concept, in which theory and reality, research and application, teaching and demonstration are all spokes of a single wheel. The success of Rush, Rochester, and their fellow experimenters should be followed closely; the outcome of their efforts could be the single most crucial turning point in American nursing history.

The Immediate Future for Nursing Roles

Although longitudinal study and rigorous, objective evaluation are the only way to assess the unification model for the development of nurse role expectations, there is much that should be done in both educational and care settings for the improvement of professional nursing. Roles need to be differentiated—perhaps never to the degree of specialization that has obtained in medicine—but nursing can no longer maintain that generic nursing is equally applicable to all fields of client needs, episodic or distributive. Joint, collaborative arrangements with medicine must be pursued to clarify and make rational the division of labor between these two vital care providers. And interim steps can be taken productively to develop conceptual schemes for the expansion and definition of role levels for nurse practitioners within the current institutions and facilities for care. Only when patients, other nurses, physicians, and administrators see nurses assuming responsibility and accepting accountability for an enlarged scope of professional conduct will they be ready to negotiate the next step and the next and the next. The unification model might provide a brilliant breakthrough; meanwhile, progress lies in the steady growth of knowledge, demonstration of clinical excellence, and professional participation in meeting the myriad demands for health care delivery. Full partnerhood, parity, equality are going to be achieved only through demonstrated capacity to contribute —and clinical excellence is the sine qua non to acceptance as a full profession. No other group has been able to avoid that responsibility; nursing must meet the same standards for acceptance.

LEADERSHIP FOR NURSING PRACTICE

One of the perplexing problems that confronted the National Commission a decade ago involved the matter of leadership for nursing practice. It was obvious that directors of nursing service played a key role in hospitals, nursing homes, and other care facilities. The nature of that role, however, was often subject to debate. Many observers argued that the director of nursing service was, in fact, more an associate hospital administrator than a chief of clinical nursing services. This view was borne out by a succession of studies and surveys that showed that movement up the administrative hierarchy in traditional settings inevitably reduced the individual's involvement in direct patient care and increased the functions associated with institutional operations.

To the extent that some individuals might wish to pursue careers in health administration, this was an entirely acceptable route. To confuse health administration with the direction of clinical services, however, was another thing entirely. Historically, there is little dispute about the fact that nurses were needed to fill those positions that in business or industry might be described as middle management roles. As the Commission on Education for Health Administration observed in 1974, "fewer than 25 per cent of executive level positions in the health and medical care system are filled by individuals who have had formal entry-level education in health administration" [24]. By extrapolation, it would seem that fewer than 5 percent of the middle-level positions in health administration could possibly be filled by prepared individuals, hence the reliance on nurses to fill in and take over many of the operational aspects of the care facility.

Along with the development of graduate training for nurses in education to meet the need for faculty came graduate preparation in administration to meet the need for managers in care facilities. Just as many educators became divorced from clinical concerns, so, too, did those nurses who followed the route of administrative promotion. For a dean or a director of nursing service to be actively involved in care decisions and clinical role modeling required a truly fierce determination to maintain currency and assume burdens added to an already formidable list of job responsibilities. Inevitably, it seemed, the administrative and managerial dimensions won out. There were exceptions, but very few.

Since 1968, however, there would seem to be growing indications that the tide is shifting. The trends in enrollment in master's and doctoral programs have shifted upward in significant increments (see Figure 4–5). Within the master's programs, the major growth has been in clinical areas of specialization and there has been a

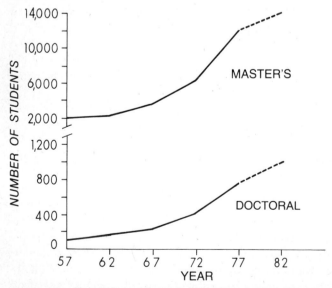

Figure 4–5   Trends in enrollment in master's and doctoral programs in nursing. *(Original artwork developed from data provided by ANA and NLN together with projections made by our study staff.)*

sharp decline in both the number and the proportion of individuals seeking administrative preparation. This means that "leadership" in nursing is more and more being defined as clinical competence at an advanced level of knowledge and skill. This trend is consistent with both the demand for increased care delivery and the reformulation of nursing roles for practice in both episodic and distributive care. The new clinical specialist or practitioner-teacher is prepared quite differently from the nurse supervisor or administrator of 1968.

At the same time, the Commission on Education for Health Administration (CEHA) and several other groups have taken up seriously the problems of preparation for executive and middle-level management positions throughout the health care system. It is perhaps an indication of the changing times that no director of nursing service served on that commission or on its panel of educational consultants. Only a few years ago, this would have seemed an egregious oversight to many people. Today, it seems like a necessary recognition of the distinction between clinical leadership and administrative initiatives. If nurses feel bad about these developments, perhaps they can take solace in the fact that earlier generations felt only physicians could be hospital administrators—physicians and executives have probably both prospered with the shift of duties.

It is important to underscore the point that clinical leaders should and must be involved in decisions related to patient care. In the same way, however, that a physician need not participate in planning alternative schemes for laundry services, clinical leaders in nursing need not be involved in the daily routines of housekeeping, supplies, and nonnursing personnel. Only when any of these operations, using the rule of the exception, disturbs patient care should nurse clinicians become involved.

On the horizon, it is possible to project the steady shift of administrative functions from nursing service to a growing cadre of middle-level health supervisors, with a concomitant increase in emphasis on clinical skills and role development throughout nursing service. In the meanwhile, there will be an extended state of flux, with traditional nursing service directors coping with staffs prepared in nontraditional ways and nurses who wish to serve essentially as clinical directors needing to establish new relationships with hospital executives and other administrative personnel.

Related to the reformulation of the role expectations and job functioning of nursing service administrators, the National Commission argued that nurses, particularly those with clinical responsibilities, should be systematically included in planning for health service agencies, patient care audits, quality assurance committees, and other activities related to the professional evolution of an expanded partnership in health care delivery. At the state level, our survey of state nurses' associations indicated that nurses were more involved in statewide activities than ever before, although many respondents felt that nurses were still designated in a spirit of tokenism. Ten state nurses' associations, however, singled out statewide health planning as the most significant area of impact that nursing had in influencing the future of health care delivery. Perhaps the clearest portrayal of how far nursing must go to achieve parity in leadership for planning and delivery of care is seen in the qualitative data on the composition of the governing boards of the 204 Health

Service Agencies reported by the Department of Health, Education, and Welfare [25]. Of the 3000 providers who served on these boards, health care institutions represented 31 percent of the total, physicians comprised 22 percent, other allied health professionals totaled 8 percent, and nurses provided 6 percent of the membership.

One of the reasons, of course, is that too many people feel a hospital or nursing home subsumes nursing interests or that medicine is representative of all clinical concerns. All the more impetus, then, for nursing to carve a clearer path for leadership in clinical, rather than institutional, concerns and to work energetically with medicine in joint practice committees to define congruent, interdependent, and independent role expectations and functions.

A final point to be made in terms of emergent leadership in nursing practice relates to the growing number of doctorally prepared nurses indicated on Figure 4–5. With approximately 20 programs for nurse-doctorates operating or announced for imminent opening, it is important to note that an increasing number and percentage of these are preparing their graduates for roles in clinical research with advanced levels of knowledge and skill in the care component. Even as the surge of master's graduates from clinical programs has spurred the development of new and deepened role expectations for nursing practice, so can the new breed of nurse doctorate holders provide important new dimensions to the redirection of nursing service administration. Prepared not as managers but as clinicians and evaluators of patient care, these individuals can supply the resources to make the unification model of full professional nursing an operational concept in more than a few demonstration sites. The impact, however, will be felt only over time. For the next decade, the organizations and societies for nursing administration must prepare the way for the next generation of leaders by moving toward greater clinical involvement and responsibility, by systematically divesting nonnursing functions, and by forcefully striving to enlarge the impact of nursing practice on the planning of the emergent health care delivery service.

TECHNOLOGY AND CHANGING SYSTEMS

In 1968, it was possible to predict that increased technology both in aspects of care and in processing of information would have profound effects upon the roles and practice of nursing. What was undefinable was the overall impact of these changes. No one would wish to do anything but advance the contributions of technology to patient care. Improved prosthetics, complex surgical interventions, advanced epidemiological techniques not only were good in themselves, but also pushed back farther and farther the boundaries of knowledge.

Information processing and retrieval, particularly through the computerization of patient records and data, can now provide visual analyses of progress and management. Nursing service not only has attacked the mundane (though very real) problems of scheduling and personnel accounting through information processing, but also has sought to analyze the intersection of client care needs and clinical competencies to assure quality care that is economically dispensed. Reanalysis of records in terms of audit programs permits a certain amount of second-guessing free from the constraints of the immediate need for critical decision making, thus improving the probabilities for better choices in the future.

Nursing service has maintained an open-mindedness toward new techniques and technology that has been characteristic of the profession over the past 50 years. Whether it is the administration of new medications, or the adoption of such new procedures as venipuncture, or the installation of a complex processing system for examination of patient management, nursing has responded affirmatively when the implications for improved patient care have been explored and evaluated. Nursing has not remained, however, a neutral cipher in this panorama of innovation and technological advance. The responsibilities of nursing have included both translating these new departures into the human terms of the patient and then dealing with the ethical and values problems that frequently accompany scientific breakthroughs.

In 1970, the National Commission observed that:

> Mass innoculations, large efforts at screening, vast educational programs all have merit and relevance. However, it is in the intimacy and immediacy of individual problems that we shall maintain—or lose—the viability of our system. On the nurse rests a major portion of the ultimate responsibility for seeing that health care is dispensed with dignity and concern [26].

If possible, this study staff should like to reiterate that observation a thousand fold. In a world and in a nation where the person often seems insignificant and powerless, where groups and blocs sometimes overshadow the individual, the need for personal, singular attention is important. In the face of acute pain and trauma, it is essential.

More eloquent than anything we could say about the necessity for nursing to continue its concern for the human element is the commentary by one physician on the care he received in a coronary unit after he had suffered a myocardial infarction. C. Henry Kempe, M.D., wrote in part of his experience at Bellevue Hospital:

> The nurses would explain what they called "scary dreams" and thus reassure me about the frequency of hallucinations . . . and that I was neither stupid nor going crazy. During those days the repeated reassurance about regaining intelligence and sanity was perhaps the most important event of the daily nursing contact. . . . The nurses taught me to ring the bell as soon as I had a bad dream. They would then turn on the light and hold my hand [27].

If an experienced and eminent physician reacts in these ways, how can we expect the less knowledgeable and the weaker to cope? In our effort to expand the scientific basis of nursing practice, we must never lose sight of what Nightingale called the *art of nursing,* that quality of human behavior that provides understanding, empathy, and support for other persons when they need it most. Physicians, other health professionals, and institutional staff personnel all share responsibility for maintaining a human system of health care and delivery. In terms of sheer numbers, presence, and role expectations, however, nurses must assume responsibility for a large proportion of the individual needs that patients have. Care with concern is the epitome of professional nursing.

In all our site visits, interviews, and surveys, there was no indication that nurse-patient relationships have faltered over the past decade. Individual complaints and anecdotal shortcomings can always be found, but the acceptance that is generally reported by patients in reaction to the enlarged scope of nursing practice and the confidence they feel is a result, in significant part, of the personal relationship between the nurse and the patient, which individualizes the therapeutic regimen and makes the client the center, rather than the periphery, of the entire system. For all our sakes, this relationship must be maintained.

The growth of our knowledge systems and the correspondent increase in technological intervention has also raised an increasing number of ethical questions for nurses and physicians. Life support systems, for example, have prolonged the survival of individuals who a few years ago might have died very quickly. The ethics of transplants, abortions, definition of death, and other issues are with us—and they do not exempt nurses from personal and professional responsibility. The increase of debate and litigation in this area has been accompanied by a growth in nurse activism. Publications on values clarification and ethical problem solving have appeared, as have increasing numbers of seminars, courses, and discussion groups.

The very nature of the concern precludes any single simplistic solution, but the need for professional consideration and movement on these issues is essential. Of course, the individual must make the final, personal commitment. In doing so, however, the nurse deserves the help and the support of peers and colleagues and, above all, the sustaining commitment of the profession itself.

The future practice patterns of nursing are still evolving. For certain, they will include greater diversification and broader expansion than we have known in the past. They will include greater science and greater art—particularly in caring. This requires greater personal responsibility and accountability, greater knowledge and conceptual ability. It will eventually end in greater risk taking and more poignant personal issues. If nurses are willing to accept this risk in return for full partnerhood and parity in the delivery of health care, they have every reason to view themselves as a true profession—and will be accepted as such. Ultimately, these movements will be anchored in collaborative joint practice with medicine and with the unification of nursing education and service in a systematic whole. For the meanwhile, however, research and innovation are essential to the development of a corpus of knowledge that can guide new roles and levels of practice in diverse settings. Perhaps the only thing for nursing to fear is reliance on traditional patterns and comfortable arrangements. For fully professional nursing, the past indeed must be prologue.

REFERENCES

1   Jerome P. Lysaught, *An Abstract for Action,* McGraw-Hill Book Company, New York, 1970, p. 11.
2   "Rating the Job of the RN," *Health Care Horizons* 2(12):1, 9 (June 17, 1979).

3 A. Flexner, *Medical Education in the United States and Canada,* D. B. Updike, The Merrymount Press, Boston, 1960.

4 Personal communication from Marian L. Rippy, executive assistant, American Nurses' Foundation to Mary Ann Christ, dated April 24, 1978.

5 Lucille E. Notter and Audrey F. Spector, *Nursing Research in the South: A Survey,* part 1, Southern Regional Education Board, Atlanta, 1974.

6 Carol Lindeman, "Priorities in Clinical Nursing Research," *Nursing Outlook* 23:693 (1975).

7 Marilyn Oberst, "Priorities in Cancer Nursing Research," *Cancer Nursing* 1(4):281–290 (August 1978).

8 Mary Ann Christ, "Research Priorities in a Nursing Unification Model," abstract of a proposal for a doctoral dissertation at The University of Rochester, Rochester, N.Y., 1978.

9 Karen B. Haller, Margaret A. Reynolds, and Jo Anne Horsley, "Developing Research-Based Innovation Protocols: Process, Criteria, and Issues," *Research in Nursing and Health* 2:45–51 (1979).

10 Personal communication from Carol A. Lindeman to Jerome P. Lysaught, dated October 5, 1979.

11 Luther Christman, "Experiment to Test and Implement a Model of Patient Care in Hospitals," in J. P. Lysaught (ed.), *A Luther Christman Anthology,* Contemporary Publications, Wakefield, Mass., 1978, pp. 50–52.

12 J. P. Lysaught, "The National Joint Practice Commission: New Bottles, New Wine," in J. P. Lysaught (ed.), *Action in Nursing: Progress in Professional Purpose,* McGraw-Hill Book Company, New York, 1974.

13 *Together: A Casebook of Joint Practices in Primary Care,* The National Joint Practice Commission, Chicago, 1977.

14 Jerome P. Lysaught, Mary Ann Christ, and Gloria Hagopian, "Progress in Professional Service: Nurse Leaders Queried," *Hospitals* 52:93ff, (August 16, 1978).

15 "The Graduate Education of Physicians," *The Report of the Citizens Commission on Graduate Medical Education,* American Medical Association, Chicago, 1966, p. 86.

16 Jerome P. Lysaught, *From Abstract into Action,* McGraw-Hill Book Company, New York, 1974, pp. 112–125.

17 "Definitions of Nursing Titles," *Nursing Practice Resource,* no. 4, The Nurses' Association of the American College of Obstetricians and Gynecologists, April 1979.

18 Rozella Schlotfeldt and Janetta MacPhail, "An Experiment in Nursing: Introducing Planned Change," *American Journal of Nursing* 69(6):1247–1251 (June 1969).

19 Ibid.

20 Luther P. Christman, "The Practitioner-Teacher: A Working Paper," unpublished manuscript, Rush University of the Health Sciences, Chicago, dated December 1973 (mimeographed).

21 Marjorie J. Powers, "The Unification Model in Nursing," *Nursing Outlook* 24:482 (1976).

22 *Nursing School Environments Inventory,* National Commission for the Study of Nursing and Nursing Education, 1968; available from Jerome P. Lysaught, University of Rochester, Rochester, N.Y.

23 Luther P. Christman, "A Micro-Analysis of the Nursing Division of One Medical Center (Rush–Presbyterian–St. Luke's Medical Center)," in Michael Millman (ed.), *Nursing*

Personnel and the Changing Health Care System, Ballinger Publishing Company, Cambridge, Mass., 1979.
24 *Summary of the Report of the Commission on Education for Health Administration,* Health Administration Press, Ann Arbor, 1974.
25 "The Purposes and Politics of HSAs," Public Affairs Advisory, National League for Nursing, New York, July 1979.
26 Lysaught, *An Abstract for Action,* p. 98.
27 C. Henry Kempe, "Nursing in a Coronary Care Unit: A Doctor-Patient's View," *The Pharos,* Winter 1979, p. 18.

Chapter 5

Implementation of the Recommendations for Nursing Education

In 1967, when the staff of the National Commission first began to collect data on the problems, needs, and resources of American nursing education, a bitter controversy was in full swing over a position paper adopted by the American Nurses' Association (ANA) House of Delegates in 1964 and published in official format the following year [1]. The two principal recommendations embodied in this document were (1) to place all nursing education in collegiate institutions and to close noncollegiate preparatory programs and (2) to distinguish between *professional* and *technical* planes of nursing, the former to be baccalaureate graduates and the latter to be prepared at the associate degree level.

Despite the fact that the first recommendation was clearly consistent with the findings and proposals of every national study of nursing education in America since 1923 [2], the negative reaction from many nurses—and from some hospital administrators and physicians—was immediate and bitter. Anger and acrimony escalated overnight. The Council of Diploma Programs of the National League for Nursing (NLN) was energized to protect the self-interest of its member institutions, and in 1965 secured the passage of a resolution by the NLN board supporting the retention of all league-accredited programs, collegiate and noncollegiate [3]. Mere defense of the status quo was insufficient for some leaders in the cause of hospital schools of nursing, and a new and militant organizational body was formed within the American Hospital Association (AHA) to perpetuate and enhance these institutions. Extremism became commonplace, and the voices of moderates were often lost in the frenzy of attack and counterattack.

At the same time, however, the second recommendation of the ANA position paper proved to be quite as disruptive to the relationship between and among the collegiate institutions for preparatory nursing education. By assigning the terms *technical* and *professional* to the 2- and 4-year programs, respectively, and using as a rationale for this division the supposed inherent and intrinsic differences between the two, the American Nurses' Association appeared to accept the view of some educators who argued that the associate degree programs were terminal in nature and wholly distinct from the professional preparatory sequence—a conceptual approach strongly rejected by many community and junior college educators and administrators.

As one acute observer put it: "For close to five decades, we've been arguing about the best way to prepare a nurse. . . . Perhaps the most concrete measure of our progress is that we are now divided into three factions instead of two. No longer is hostility concentrated between the collegiate and the hospital-based program . . . it's now split three ways" [4].

Several state nurses' associations attempted to develop blueprints for implementing the position paper, but resistance from hospital schools and lack of acceptance by associate degree programs proved to be formidable obstacles. In addition, a number of educational directors and faculty from baccalaureate and higher degree programs expressed their misgivings and reservations about aspects of the position paper and its recommendations. Some felt that articulation between the two levels of collegiate preparation was possible and desirable; in some states where the lower- and upper-division pattern for public institutions of higher education was established, it might even be legally required. A few innovative educators felt that the traditional parameters of baccalaureate nursing education were, in themselves, a constraint that the position paper did not address. Still others felt that the entire argument about *professional* and *technical* levels of nursing turned on assertions that had no actual basis in research findings or hard data [5].

It was in this atmosphere of confusion, distrust, and downright antagonism that the National Commission set out to develop an independent and objective analysis of American nursing education and the rationale for a system of cooperating units that would combine to provide excellence in learning *along with* access to individual and career options. To develop a comprehensive and congruent pattern for nursing education in this country, the Commission became convinced that the collegiate system was the only viable pathway. On reaching this conclusion, however, the staff was charged with the task of developing a variety of plans and suggestions for making such a transition both positive and progressive, reducing the level of discord and harshness. If the noncollegiate institutions were to be replaced, it was understood that there must be related changes in *both* 2-year and 4-year institutions so that an articulated, interdigitated, and jointly planned *collegiate system* might emerge. In order to meet the needs of individual nurses and the profession at large, the Commission called for a "spirit of cooperative concern" to replace the emotionalism and strident partisanship that had characterized so many earlier attempts at change and redirection.

Over the period from 1970 through 1973, the Commission and its staff worked with educators and administrators from all varieties of preparatory programs to effect the objectives outlined in *An Abstract for Action*. Substantial progress was made at the institutional level and in the creation of statewide planning activities designed to facilitate interinstitutional cooperation and provide better and longer perspectives on needs, problems, and resources. No one could be sanguine over the enormous task of dealing with more than 1300 programs in 51 separate legal and political jurisdictions, but a start could be made. And it was.

Following the termination of the formal implementation phase of the National Commission, in 1973, and prior to the initiation of this longitudinal assessment, in 1978, one unanticipated variable appeared which may have a tremendous impact on the development of an educational system for nursing in the United States. At the 1978 biennial meeting of the American Nurses' Association, the House of Delegates adopted what is commonly referred to as the *1985 resolution*. This would go beyond the 1965 position paper in several significant aspects. First, it would place all professional nursing education within the collegiate system, and it would designate the baccalaureate degree as the base for entry into the profession by 1985. Second, it would designate graduates of associate degree and diploma programs, after 1985, as *nurse associates* with separate licensure or certification at a nonprofessional level. Third, to assist in establishing such an educational pattern, national guidelines are to be formulated and a comprehensive prescription is to be written listing the behavioral competencies appropriate to each of the two levels of nursing practice— professional and associate. Finally, there would be provision, up to 1985, for "grand-fathering" all those registered nurses licensed before the cutoff date into the classifi-cation of professional nurse since there is currently no legal distinction in any state on a licensing examination among graduates of associate degree, diploma, and baccalaureate preparatory programs.

The ANA delegates and the resolution speak to the importance of quality programs for career mobility, but it would appear that the legal separation of *professional* nursing from *associate* nursing would have far more sweeping conse-quences for the articulation of 2- and 4-year programs than the previous proposals to categorize graduates of the different programs as either professional or technical while retaining one common examination for safe practice and licensure.

One predictable consequence of the 1985 resolution is that the atmosphere of discussion about nursing education will once more be charged with acrimony and suspicion [6]. Advocates endorse the proposal as a natural step in the developmental effort to upgrade the profession; some acerbic critics view the resolution as one more evidence of a raw grab for power by baccalaureate nurse educators and their support-ers. For everyone involved in or affected by nursing education, the resolution pro-vides a dramatic challenge to the concepts of access, affirmative action, articulation, and career mobility.

In the face of hardening lines and heightening emotion, the need for intelligent and empathic leadership was never greater in American nursing. There is, however, a paucity of time. If no consensus or compromise can be reached on the systems and patterns for nursing education by the end of 1980, then there is little likelihood that the profession will be able to solve the unremitting problem of a bifurcated educational system before the end of the century. For more than 75 years, nursing has lived with and suffered from a "nonsystem" of education. Today, there are an increasing number of external agencies and bodies that are ready, willing, and legally capable of imposing solutions that are unlikely to please any of the protagonists within the nursing profession [7]. The question, very simply, is whether nursing will make a decision that will effect harmony from within or someone else will make a determination from without—not to act is also a decision, not to act in the face of evident need and external threat is an abdication of professional responsibility.

In reviewing the progress on the recommendations of the National Commission for the Study of Nursing and Nursing Education (NCSNNE), this staff conducted a series of on-site visits to educational institutions and consortia; surveyed national samples of students, deans, and directors; and systematically queried or interviewed state nurses' associations, constituent leagues, regional planning groups for nursing education, and a variety of national, state, and local groups. Over the next several sections, we hope to present a current picture of status, accomplishment, and failings as well as suggestions for "next steps" toward the establishment of an articulated and effective system for American nursing education. In presenting this analysis, the material will be treated in the same order of presentation as were the eight areas of recommendations presented in *An Abstract for Action.*

INSTITUTIONAL PATTERNS FOR NURSING EDUCATION

In her report on the first national study of nursing in the United States, Josephine Goldmark observed that the hospital training schools did not conform to the standards accepted—and required—in other educational fields [8]. The year was 1923. A periodic series of studies over the next 40 years corroborated this finding and, without exception, recommended that nursing education be placed within the collegiate mainstream of American higher education while retaining its historic ties to the hospital through use of hospital facilities as a site for clinical training and experience [9]. Thus the American Nurses' Association position paper of 1965 in its call for an all-collegiate pattern for registered nurse education was unique only in its insistence that there be proximate action to fulfill that recommendation. The response to this proposal, however, was remarkable in its intensity among program directors and administrators who were committed to the maintenance of hospital schools of nursing—without reservation, qualification, or compromise.

The ensuing and continuing argument over the loci of nursing education is all the more remarkable when we view it in the light of other professions' experience. In 1910, at the time the Flexner report was disseminated, the majority of medical schools in the United States were free-standing, proprietary institutions. In less than three decades, these "independent" medical training schools were almost wholly replaced by university-related medical colleges, with a strong foundation in the basic sciences and research methods as an entree into clinical training. Over almost this same time period, professional education moved from a prevalent pattern of public "noncollegiate" normal schools in 1900 to the development, first, of teacher's colleges and, then, of professional departments or schools located within a full university setting. Proprietary, didactic schools of medicine disappeared; pedantic, circumscribed normal schools for teachers disappeared; noncollegiate hospital training schools for nurses continued, even though their numbers were sharply reduced over time.

In 1970, the National Commission for the Study of Nursing and Nursing Education endorsed the proposition that all nursing education should be placed in the mainstream of American collegiate education and that its preparatory programs should be housed in the 2- and 4-year colleges. Unlike the earlier proposals for closing out the hospital schools, which essentially gave no direction or timetable for such a terminal operation, the Commission proposed a set of alternatives for consideration by these institutions as well as a process for determining realistic deadlines for conversion and adjustment.

Those hospital schools that were academically distinguished and financially endowed were encouraged to seek regional and state accreditation as collegiate institutions in their own right, with degree-granting power. A number of institutions, some singly, some on a cooperative basis, have indeed pursued this approach to a successful conclusion [10]. Still others are in the process of documenting their qualifications and resources. Although this alternative was recognized as a sharply limited choice, it nevertheless was a viable and proper goal for a number of distinguished institutions, and the fact that some hospitals schools have been transformed into colleges underscores the need for careful assessment on an institution-by-institution basis and the avoidance of broad and uncritical generalization.

Most of the hospital schools of nursing were encouraged to move quickly and systematically to effect cooperative arrangements with collegiate institutions so that joint assessment of strengths and resources could be accomplished. The collegiate institution would take responsibility for the academic program, and the hospital could provide enhanced clinical settings and, often, a number of well-qualified faculty persons who could serve with distinction in the teaching of patient care. The hospital would continue to have students within its wards and units and an opportunity to attract and recruit individuals who had practiced in that setting. The college would gain both physical and human resources. The students, while pursuing a degree program with enhanced access to advanced and graduate education, would experience an optimum arrangement of didactic instruction and clinical preparation. The development could provide benefits to all concerned—the institutions, the faculty, and, above all, the students.

A small number of hospital schools, those that were particularly weak and located in areas where openings for nursing students were in abundance, were counseled to close their programs as quickly as possible—but always with advanced planning and notification to the adjacent institutions. Even here, the possibility remained that clincial facilities within the hospital could be used to enhance the educational program of a nearby college. Through the replacement of competition by institutional cooperation, there could be a new growth of structural patterning in nursing education that would accomplish the goals envisaged by the Commission for the 1980s: a collegiate system of nursing education that would provide multiple entry, upward mobility, institutional articulation, and predictable routes of access for future generations of students.

A Concept of Nursing Education Systems

In order to provide the capabilities specified for a new system of nursing education, the National Commission developed a conceptual scheme (Figure 5–1) that would significantly change the traditional form of institutions and their relationships. The noncollegiate schools would disappear, but access would be assured for the thousands of graduates of diploma schools who would require entry to and mobility within the system. In this plan, there would be four general routes to the Bachelor of Science degree in nursing:

   1   The generic 4-year program would be retained; this program would consist generally of 2 years of general arts and science followed by preparatory courses in nursing science and clinical intervention.
   2   A simple variation would consist of interinstitutional arrangements such that associate degree students could fulfill the prenursing requirements within a lower-division institution and transfer into the nursing sequence upon completion of their program.
   3   A more innovative approach would be the development of a two-plus-two arrangement in which an upper division program in nursing *and* related disciplines would be planned to build upon the base provided by the associate degree in nursing that also included both nursing and nonnursing components.
   4   The programs designed to accomplish the articulation of A.D.N. and B.S.N. programs could also facilitate the entry of diploma school graduates into the collegiate system. For those with some academic deficiencies in the nonnursing areas, the associate degree institution might be the one to facilitate the completion of prerequisites. For those who have met these basics, the upper-division baccalaureate program can provide clinical and didactic opportunities in nursing which build on the experience of these registered nurses.

Still an additional option is afforded by a fifth route that provides articulation for those licensed practical or vocational nurses who wish to pursue the goal of becoming registered nurses. The conceptual scheme proposed here would anticipate that the L.P.N. program would be of collegiate caliber and would be generally patterned after the competencies developed in the first year of an associate degree program in registered nursing.

As a guarantee that this conceptual approach to a varied but harmonious system for nursing education is not mere fancy, but is both practical and meritorious, every one of its facets has been subjected to analysis, development, and evaluation by the Orange County/Long Beach Consortium for Nursing Education since 1972 [11]. Although the requirements for interinstitutional planning and cooperation are demanding, it is possible for associate, baccalaureate, and graduate institutions to develop interlocking goals and objectives such that exit competencies from one

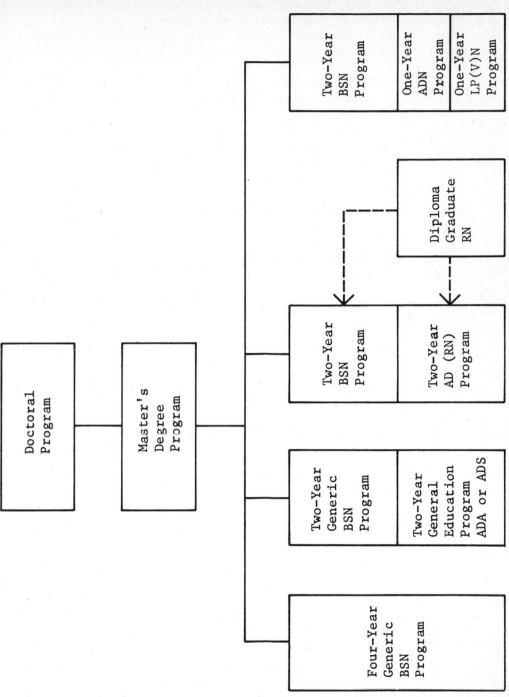

Figure 5-1 Schematic representation of a multiple-entry, articulated system for nursing education in the United States.

program become entrance expectations for the succeeding level—and so on. Likewise, it is possible for students to exit from the system at various points to accept employment with the assurance that their reentry can be facilitated and appropriately managed.

There is no attempt in this schema to erect a monolithic pathway, nor is there any effort to require all institutions to provide all varieties of instructional programming. Rather, this approach encourages institutional diversity, coupled with interinstitutional planning and cooperation. It is precisely because our present institutions and configurations do not accommodate themselves well to the realities of the situation that we must adopt new and imaginative approaches to the preparation of our student nurses. It could be argued that any system would be superior to our nonsystem; through planning, cooperation, and articulation, it is possible to improve every element in the pattern so that the whole is qualitatively better than any one of the parts that we utilize today.

Statewide Master Planning Committees

The Commission strongly believed in a national pattern for future nursing education and for regional planning and development of undergraduate and graduate programming, but the control of education is constitutionally reserved to the states. This fact, coupled with related licensure and practice acts, made it necessary that the implementation process be taken up in each of the 51 jurisdictions involved.

To effect changes in the education system and to provide objectivity and continuity in the implementation process, it was recommended that each state establish a statewide master planning committee that would include representatives of nursing, other health professions, and the public to develop specific guidelines, goals and objectives, and timetables to bring about a comprehensive collegiate system for nursing education. There should be uniformity in the terminal competencies expected of beginning practitioners (at least in respect to their ability to successfully pass a general licensure examination), but there should be opportunity for a wide diversity in ways and means for obtaining those competencies.

Over the period from 1970 through 1973, the Commission's staff and regional advisers worked with state nurses' association, health planning groups, departments of higher education, legislative bodies, and other appropriate agencies to establish statewide master planning committees. Early on, it became apparent that some general guidelines might be useful, but each of the states possessed unique attributes, needs, and resources that dictated a highly individualized approach. The location of the committee, for instance, and its composition had to take into account the governmental features and historic experience of the many jurisdictions. Neglect of or transgressions upon unique characteristics inevitably resulted in problems and delays.

Careful efforts were made to maintain records on the establishment and activities of the statewide master planning committees through the close of the formal implementation period in 1973. In the course of this longitudinal survey, the state nurses' associations were asked to report on the current status of these bodies and to comment on their activities. Table 5–1 displays the comparative status of state planning committees for 3 years: in 1971, at the close of 1 year of national implemen-

Table 5-1   Number and Percentage of State Master Planning Committees Established in the United States, 1971–1978

Year	Number of state master planning committees	Percentage*
1971	11	22
1973	26	51
1978	32	63

*The percentage is based on 51 jurisdictions, the 50 states and the District of Columbia.

tation; in 1973, at the close of 3 years of national implementation; and in 1978, five years after the closing of national implementation. The figures show a continuing increase in establishment and activation; three times as many states possessed a master planning committee in 1978 as did in 1971. The pace of establishment has slowed considerably, and much more remains to be done. In the 5-year period from 1973 through 1978, there was a gain of only six statewide groups; taken all together, we reached 63 percent of the total goal.

In the 19 states that were still without a statewide master planning committee, nursing education was planned and monitored by a broad variety of agencies, with significant differences in completeness and success. In some instances, state boards of education were assigned this function; in other cases, the state board of nursing was the primary agency for planning and regulation. The relationship of professional nursing organizations to these governing bodies varied from strong involvement through intermittent discussion to an almost adversary position. Frequently, the control of 2- and 4-year programs and the direction of public and private institutions was fragmented and no single agency or authority had full responsibility.

The need for a designated, representative, and objective body seems, however, to be broadly accepted. At this time, three more states—Kentucky, Arkansas, and Georgia—are seeking to implement the establishment of a statewide master planning committee. Two others, Wisconsin and New Hampshire, have completed their planning and developmental processes and are moving on toward the enactment of their recommendations. The addition of these five states to our active bodies would bring us to the 73 percent level in terms of implementing the recommendations of the National Commission.

Although there is satisfaction, then, in the continuing growth and development of statewide master planning committees, it must be recognized that one out of every four states has still not moved aggressively toward the planning of an educational system for nursing that can solve the accumulated problems of the past 60 years. Our agenda can never be completed until every state has developed guidelines and deadlines for the reconstruction of its educational patterns for nursing preparation. Much has been done; more remains to be accomplished.

Hospital Schools of Nursing

Shortly after the appearance of the National Commission's recommendations on nursing education, the Council of Diploma Programs of the National League for Nursing voted its nonsupport of the proposal to establish a collegiate system of nursing education and, of course, of any implementation efforts directed toward such a goal. The more vociferous Assembly of Hospital Schools of Nursing of the American Hospital Association resolved to "repudiate any individuals or groups who 'alluded' to the phasing out of diploma programs for nursing education." Neither group made mention in its rhetoric that every national study of nursing since 1923 had independently come to the same conclusion and recommendation—that only a collegiate system of education could effectively, efficiently, and qualitatively meet the long-range needs of the profession. The reasoning behind this recommendation is well ordered and documented; the attempts at refutation are riddled with emotionalism, self-serving platitudes, and a refusal to look at the outcomes of a bifurcated preparatory arrangement [12].

Having anticipated that such organizational posturing would be forthcoming, the Commission and its staff were not surprised. As a matter of fact, it was hoped that some "organizational ventilation" might be useful in developing a more sensitive, sensible synthesis to the problem once the immediate anger had subsided. For 3 years, 1970 through 1973, the staff worked with individual hospital schools and with the national associations to gain an understanding of the recommendations *and* of the alternatives that might be invoked to unlock the status quo. Statewide master planning committees lent their encouragement to the development of a collegiate system, and an increasing number of individual nurses took leadership roles in exploring ways to integrate their institutions into a new pattern and system for nursing education [13].

As indicated in Table 5-2, the decline in the number of diploma programs was significantly accelerated over the period from 1968 to 1973—years that coincide with the distribution of the National Commission's preliminary findings and recommendations through the conclusion of its formal implementation activities. More to the point, however, there were 636 hospital schools of nursing in 1970, when *An Abstract for Action* appeared; in 1974, at the end of the implementation period, there were only 460 programs still in existence—a decrease of some 28 percent. No one agency or organization was responsible for this effect, but there is no doubt that the recommendations of the Commission lent credence and urgency to the need to reexamine educational processes in nursing.

Table 5-2   Number of Hospital School Diploma Programs and Admissions in the United States, 1953–1978

Year	Number of diploma programs	Admissions
1953	926	36,000*
1958	920	37,457
1963	857	37,571
1968	727	28,971
1973	493	26,943
1978	344	20,611

*Figures for 1953 are rounded estimates based on data presented in *Nursing Outlook*, September 1978, p. 573.

Many of the 176 programs that closed between 1970 and 1974 were small in size and resources. Taken all together, they accounted for relatively small shifts in total diploma student admissions and graduations. The decline in admissions to diploma schools, for example, was only 14 percent for this period, emphasizing the fact that the larger and stronger programs were continuing to operate. A strong trend, however, had been established and set in motion.

At the end of 1973, the National Commission projected that there would be a continuing decrease in the number of hospital schools and that the impact on admissions and graduations would become more apparent as the larger and more prestigious hospital schools began to phase out of existence. From 1973 through 1978, there was a further reduction in the number of diploma programs from 493 to 344, a decline of approximately 30 percent. Admissions to diploma programs continued to decrease both in actual and in relative numbers over this same period (Figure 5–2). Whereas hospital schools of nursing accounted for 57 percent of all preparatory admissions in 1966 (the year before the National Commission was established), their "share of the market" had shrunk to 20 percent in 1978. The projection for the future (Figure 5–3) is even more pronounced since it embodies the multiple effects of reduced facilities, declining enrollments, and economic pressures. If it is accurate, hospital schools, by 1985, will provide less than 10 percent of our registered nurse graduates.

More of the larger hospital schools of nursing have begun the process of effecting interinstitutional arrangements with colleges and universities. A survey of 77 hospital schools of nursing in 1978 (as part of a randomized sample of 264 preparatory institutions for nursing education) revealed that no less than 50 percent were actively involved in some stage of planning with a collegiate institution to articulate their programs and move toward a collegiate system. A few diploma

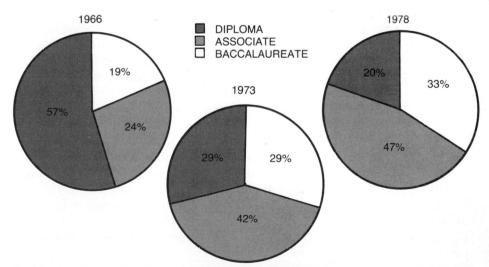

Figure 5–2 Share of admissions to diploma, associate, and baccalaureate programs, 1966–1978. *(Original artwork based on data provided by ANA and NLN.)*

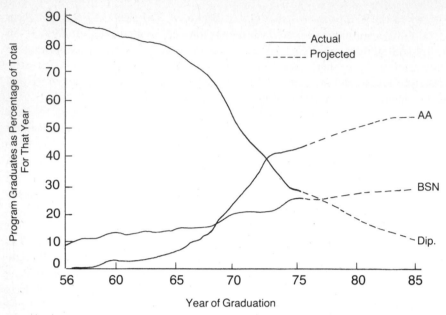

Figure 5-3 Percentage share of graduates for preparatory nursing programs, actual and projected, 1956–1985. *(From The Journal of Health Politics, Policy and Law. Copyright 1978 by the Department of Health Administration, Duke University. Used with permission.)*

schools were taking the more difficult path toward accreditation as bona fide collegiate institutions in their own right; in some cases this was being done through a cooperative effort involving the resources of more than one institution.

Some portion of the movement among hospital schools may be attributed to the rational argument, moral suasion, and direct assistance provided by the National Commission, its staff, and its advisers over the formal period of implementation, but it is difficult to separate out the particular reasons for each institutional decision. Any honest analysis would have to include the effect of the recession of 1975–1978 and the concomitant cost containment efforts of hospitals and governmental agencies. The decision by many third-party payers to eliminate support for preparatory education expenses was a dominant factor in some decisions to terminate programs. The diploma programs will continue to become more vulnerable in the months to come as the pressure mounts ever higher on hospitals to place a ceiling on expenditures unrelated to direct patient care. This movement bears out, in large part, both the Commission's analysis of actual costs of nursing education and Altman's econometric predictions on the future of diploma schools [14]. In his view, the costs of hospital schools of nursing alone will decisively end the argument in favor of a collegiate system by 1985. In the experience of the Commission, much more is required in terms of planning, negotiation, and encouragement, but the final causative factor may never be determined or isolated.

If much has been accomplished, and it has, any exuberance is tempered by a sober reassessment of the remaining problem. Currently, there are more than 340 operational diploma schools of nursing. Since the termination of the formal implementation phase, more than 80,000 individuals have completed training in a noncollegiate, hospital training program. Each one of these nurses represents another challenge to our capacity for access and mobility. Even when we look ahead to 1985, if our projections are accurate, we will still be graduating between 10,000 and 12,000 nurses per annum from hospital programs. Still more incredible is the fact that no less than two new diploma programs have been established since 1974! The direction is set; the pattern is inevitable. But it is also clear that some number of institutions will apparently never close of their own volition, and while they remain open, there will never be a *system* for nursing education.

In the light of what remains to be done, it is essential that we repeat the preeminent reason for the Commission's recommendation that there be one articulated collegiate system for nursing education:

> In summary, the Commission sees a critical need for planned change in American nursing education so that students will be given proper rewards for accomplishment, enhanced opportunities for career mobility, and broadened personal vistas throughout their lifetime of learning. Our recommendations for repatterning of education are designed specifically to accomplish this [15].

Thus, the National Commission came to its conclusions, not on the basis of institutional politics or on the premise of "professional power enhancement." The decision was based simply and surely on the documented experience of graduates from these diploma programs, their frustrations when they sought to enhance their careers, and the exorbitant costs they had to pay in order to obtain broadened access and upward mobility. No amount of rationalization can explain away the reality of our nonsystem.

Any continuing number of admissions to and graduations from these diploma schools is distressing; 81,000 persons since 1973 is unconscionable; and the several thousands more still to be caught up in this situation—so long as these institutions remain open—will be a long-lasting reminder that nursing alone, of all the emergent professions, maintains a divided and divisive system of education that militates against its own and that should have been abandoned in the early decades of the twentieth century. The testimony of the Goldmark Commission and all the years since 1923 is left to stand as a monument to the difficulty of change in educational organization for nursing.

To explain why nursing education has not completed this first step toward a reconstructed pattern of professional preparatory education is not easy. The answer lies, in large part, within the profession—in both its individuals and its institutions. No educational program in nursing could exist if nurses themselves did not provide the faculty and the administration. The remaining diploma schools of nursing would be closed overnight if nurses refused to perpetuate them. But, in truth, can individuals be singled out when national organizations support and prolong the status quo?

In February of 1971, the National League for Nursing, the accrediting body for all registered nursing programs, endorsed the summary report and recommendations of the National Commission through formal action of its Board of Directors. Immediately afterward, the Council of Diploma Programs expressed its dismay, and the board established a task force to study the implications of the Commission's proposals. The task force never met with or discussed the recommendations with the Commission or its staff. It accepted the general thrust of the recommendation concerning a collegiate system for nursing education, but the task force took upon itself the responsibility for deleting the word *deadlines* from the statement because "the implied threat of forcing institutions to close was rejected as unnecessary" [16]. History has shown just how naive this sentiment was. The National League for Nursing has assumed no forceful leadership in the development of a collegiate system for nursing education and has maintained the posture that there are and should remain three preparatory routes to the registered nurse license—hospital school, associate degree, and baccalaureate institutions [17]. No organization should have better data on the results of such a policy, but income from membership and from accreditation fees is perhaps more significant than thousands of personal problems.

Nor is the American Nurses' Association exempt from challenge on its record regarding a reformation of preparatory nursing. In 1965, the ANA called for the elimination of diploma schools. In the 1985 resolution, there is a provision for a one-time grandfathering operation but no mention of an outright effort to close the hospital schools in order to effect an all-collegiate system. In short, let the diploma schools and their students look to themselves after 1985 since they will no longer be considered part of the professional establishment. Student nurses deserve better than this, and it ill behooves the professional body that presumes to speak for all American nurses not to address the situation clearly and directly.

Currently, there are 42 percent fewer hospital schools of nursing than there were in 1970. From the indications of the longitudinal survey of these institutions, almost half of those remaining are involved in substantive discussions and planning with institutions of higher education concerning the possibility of articulation and joint activity. Moreover, in more than 60 percent—possibly as many as 75 percent —of our states, planning committees are attempting to develop a comprehensive interinstitutional pattern for collegiate nursing education. Now is the critical time for the organizations that speak for nurses and their educational institutions to make a final commitment. In 1970, it may have been argued that the time was premature, that there had been too little joint planning and interinstitutional agreement. Today, these conditions are significantly different; it is time for the National League for Nursing and the American Nurses' Association to exert the leadership they claim to possess.

An optimist reviewing the transformation of the patterning for nursing education would argue that we are halfway to our goals; a pessimist would insist that we have failed by half to reach them. An idealist would deplore the fact that more years have been consumed in the struggle to make nursing education a unified and articulated system. A realist would simply say that the hardest part of the fight is still ahead and that our efforts must be doubled and redoubled accordingly. By any measure, there is an unfinished agenda that must be addressed with determination and decisiveness. The students, in the last analysis, shall be the ones who pay for our follies or reap the benefits of our wisdom.

Collegiate Schools of Nursing

In 1970, the National Commission proposed, "To ensure that one pitfall is not substituted for another under a new pattern, we also feel that the junior and senior colleges should eliminate any needless barriers to or between their programs." Baccalaureate programs in nursing, from their very inception, had to deal with the problems of the registered nurse who had graduated from a noncollegiate diploma school and then aspired to a college degree. Even with the best of intentions, there were problems and hazards attached to such an arrangement.

With the establishment of associate degree programs in nursing in the junior and community colleges of the country, one might have hoped for a better system of articulation and upward mobility. This was not the case. Proponents of the associate degree programs initially espoused the view that these sequences were technical and terminal—and many still do today. By this, they meant that the cognitive, affective, and psychomotor skills taught in the curriculum were distinctly limited and not intended to be stepping-stones into advanced instructional programs at the baccalaureate level. They were complete in themselves, and their parameters were sharply circumscribed. One graduated from such a program as a beginning technical nurse; one did not develop the prerequisites for becoming a professional nurse.

This conceptual model was quite compatible with the belief system that other educators had constructed about baccalaureate nursing programs. To them, the ideal preparatory program, the so-called generic approach, consisted of an upper-division body of professional scientific and clinical courses built on a framework of lower-division courses in prescribed nonnursing fields: the arts, behavioral sciences, and biological sciences. Thus, the junior nursing student would have had no professional courses in his or her own discipline, but would have completed a full set of prerequisite studies in other departments. Obviously, the graduate of a 2-year college, who had already taken some nursing science courses and a different arrangement of nonnursing courses (and who quite likely had already passed the licensure examination for registration as a nurse), was, by definition, out of step in relation to an orderly progression of studies.

Generic baccalaureate nursing programs have always been under great pressure to accommodate their curricula to transfer students. Until 1970, approximately 85 percent of all baccalaureate degree nurses had first graduated from a diploma school and had been licensed as registered nurses before entering the collegiate program. With the decline of the hospital school and the emergence of associate degree programs, there has been a pronounced shift in the locus of prebaccalaureate training, but the problem is still acute. As the American Nurses' Association noted in 1978:

> WHEREAS, The overwhelming majority of registered nurses currently do not hold a baccalaureate degree in nursing . . .

THEREFORE BE IT RESOLVED THAT: ANA actively support increased accessibility to high quality career mobility programs which utilize flexible approaches for individuals seeking academic degrees in nursing [18].

With the professional emphasis on the baccalaureate degree as the entry level into nursing practice, there is a greater urgency than ever before to provide an articulated system for moving from one educational level to another. Perhaps an even stronger compulsion lies in the projections for needed nurse practitioners in 1982 prepared by the Western Interstate Commission on Higher Education (WICHE). Using the commission's lower-bound criteria, it would appear that we may have a surplus of some 332,000 diploma and associate degree nurses and a deficit of 506,000 baccalaureate nurses in the United States. Using the upper-bound criteria, the surplus of associate and diploma nurses would be reduced to 202,000, but the deficit of baccalaureate nurses would climb to 834,000 [19]. These figures, it should be emphasized, are based on estimates of client care needs, not professional prerogatives.

The point at issue is, of course, Where could 278,000 to 834,000 additional baccalaureate and graduate degreed nurses come from? The only possibility for such massive upgrading lies in the mobility potential of the associate degree and diploma nurses. Grace estimates that it would require an increase of 850 to 1000 baccalaureate programs in nursing—over and above the existing 350—to develop adequate numbers of B.S.N. students using only generic programs and institutions [20]. Such an approach is out of the realm of possibility for many reasons, cost being only one of the factors that would prevent its creation. On the other hand, the continued development of one out of every two licensed R.N.s from diploma or associate degree to the baccalaureate level would meet the lower-bound criteria of the WICHE projections, and the mobility of two out of every three R.N.s to the baccalaureate or graduate level would go a long way toward satisfying the upper-bound criteria.

As indicated in Figure 5-4, half or more of the registered nurses who are attending collegiate programs are in baccalaureate—not graduate—sequences. This situation has had two profound effects on the generic institutions: first, it has forced them constantly to compromise their curriculum because many, if not most, of their students did not fit the model for prerequisites and entry behavior; second, it has developed false expectations among many faculty and more employing agencies about the expectations for baccalaureate graduates. Most of the "post-R.N." baccalaureate students were older, more mature, more self-directed, and more work-experienced than students coming directly from secondary schools could possibly be expected to be. Nevertheless, generalizations about baccalaureate graduates too often failed to make these differentiations. All baccalaureate students were expected to be leaders—ready to step into any situation and perform as a full professional—as well as excellent practitioners.

Perhaps no other professional group in America has expected so much of its baccalaureate graduates. For most of the true generic students—those who had completed the 4-year collegiate program and had just passed the licensure examination—there was a "reality shock" of great proportions. In short, the admixture of students and the compromise in the curriculum of the baccalaureate degree pro-

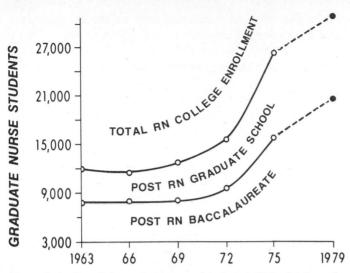

Figure 5–4   Trends in graduate nurse enrollment. Of the total enrollment of registered nurses in colleges and universities, approximately half are completing baccalaureate education and the other half are pursuing graduate studies. *(Original artwork based on data provided by ANA and NLN.)*

grams in nursing resulted in a less than optimal situation for both R.N. and generic students. It is for this reason that the National Commission proposed a variety of preparatory routes and programs designed to accommodate the known subsets of individuals with differing experiential and academic backgrounds.

Four-year generic programs should be preserved, and their curricular patterns should remain intact. They have proven their ability to recruit, admit, and graduate excellent beginning nurses with professional commitment and with the capacity for pursuing advanced clinical and educational challenges.

Registered nurses, however, should be offered opportunities for baccalaureate education in programs specifically designed for their needs, experience, and assessed entry levels. Alternative programs that preserve academic integrity while vastly increasing flexibility and access are vitally needed.

It is not any failure on the part of generic programs but, rather, the need for a companion structure within the system of collegiate nursing education which causes the emphasis by the National Commission and its staff on an alternative approach to baccalaureate education for registered nurses.

The first requirement of an integrated lower- and upper-division program for nursing education is the development of interinstitutional planning and cooperation. Curricula for the associate and baccalaureate programs need to be matched in terms of core requirements and elective concentrations—or, using other descriptors, jointly planned so as to produce agreement on universals, alternatives, and conceptual integrations. The objective should be to ensure that the levels of competencies (cognitive, affective, and psychomotor skills) for exit from the 2-year program are accepted as the entrance levels for the baccalaureate program. Such an approach was pioneered in the Orange County/Long Beach Consortium [21] and, more recently, has been refined into a taxonomy of nursing competencies by the Nursing Curriculum Project of the Southern Regional Education Board [22]. A number of "two plus two" programs have been initiated, and the first research conference on curriculum, evaluation, and related studies has been called by Sonoma State University for 1980 [23].

If the first requirement of change is interinstitutional planning and curricular organization, the essential corollary is the development of a healthy heterodoxy on the subject of how best to prepare baccalaureate nursing students. In some cases, perhaps in most, institutions should make a choice based on their own strength and resources—guided, too, by area and regional needs. In a smaller number of situations, colleges and universities may mount more than one program and still ensure quality and diversity. California State University at Long Beach has demonstrated its capacity to offer both generic and upper-division programs and to blend the students and faculty into a conceptual whole [24].

One indication of how far the "unfreezing" of the status quo has proceeded is found in the survey of a striated, random sample of deans and directors of collegiate programs in nursing completed in 1977. Fifty-six percent of the associate degree programs and 61 percent of the baccalaureate institutions reported that they had ongoing planning activities looking into the examination of curricula and interinstitutional programming for articulation. These figures strongly suggest that the concept of wholly separate education has been quietly buried by a majority of the collegiate programs for nursing and that considerable activity is taking place in the development of mechanisms and arrangements for transition between 2- and 4-year colleges.

Just as a combination of economic, social, and professional forces will ultimately decide the solution to the problems of the noncollegiate preparatory programs in nursing, so the same basic issues will determine that a multiple entry and an articulated system of collegiate preparatory programs will emerge to stand beside our traditional generic configurations. At the very least, such a transition would permit nursing to devote time to those issues that will become ever more significant to the future of the profession: graduate learning, continuing education, and expanded needs for advanced clinical training.

PROBLEMS OF PREPARATORY INSTITUTIONS

One outcome of the continuing rancor over the patterning of preparatory education has been the inability of the nursing profession to speak with one clear voice about the common needs and problems that are experienced by almost every institution that seeks to train students for entry into practice. As a result, problems begin to present an enduring quality that defies resolution. In 1968, we asked the deans and directors of all kinds of nursing preparatory programs to list in order of priority their greatest problems and needs. In 1978, Hagopian undertook a doctoral research project into the administrative problems of deans of baccalaureate and higher degree programs in nursing [25]. The results of the two inquires are displayed in Table 5–3.

Over the 10-year period between the two investigations, the matter of obtaining

Table 5-3 Comparison of Educational Problems Cited by Nurse Educational Leaders in 1968 and 1978

Problem	Priority in 1968	Priority in 1978
Faculty recruitment, development and retention	1	1
Financial support and fiscal concerns	2	2
Inadequate and outmoded facilities	3	4
Implementing change	4	3
Curriculum development and evaluation	5	5

and retaining faculty continued to be the single most frequently cited problem for the preparatory institutions. The animus between collegiate and noncollegiate programs and the lack of an open system for upward mobility had a profound impact upon the number of nurses entering the graduate programs that traditionally have served as the faculty training grounds for all other professions. The academic preparation of nurse faculty members at all institutions tended to be depressed in comparison with any other discipline or profession of comparable complexity and public service. As indicated in Figure 5-5, well over half of the faculty at our current hospital schools were prepared only through the baccalaureate, whereas the majority of all collegiate faculty members were prepared at the master's level or below. Over a period of 8 years, from 1970 to 1978, however, the proportion of master's-level faculty in baccalaureate programs increased by only 2 percent and doctorally prepared faculty by just 4 percent. Other changes could be cited in the same restricted terms. It was not that institutions had not sought to recruit more qualified people —it was simply a matter of limited supply and high demand. Indeed, the competition for doctorally prepared nursing faculty had been most intense and the demand for master's prepared faculty was far greater than for a similarly prepared individual in any of the traditional academic areas. As a consequence, turnover continued to be high; individuals found a ready marketplace bidding for their employment; and some salaries rose disproportionately to those of other academic fields.

The short-term advantages, however, may be offset by the long-term consequences. Nursing faculty, in order to obtain promotion, tenure, and continued salary advancement, must inevitably meet the general standards established for other academic disciplines and professions. Parenthetically, it has been observed that both doctorally prepared and master's prepared nurses have by dint of circumstances been all too frequently placed into positions of academic leadership (deans, department heads, etc.) for which they have had neither experience nor training. This situation has furthered the problems of retention and turnover.

Close behind the problems of faculty recruitment and development are the fiscal concerns of preparatory programs in nursing. In the mid-1950s, the Health Manpower Training Acts and the subsequent Nurse Training Acts of the 1960s repre-

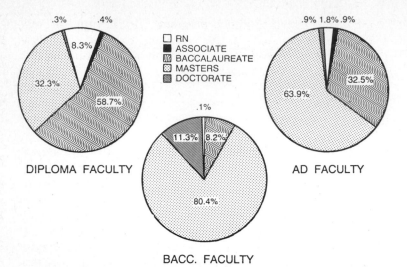

Figure 5–5   Academic preparation of nurse faculty by highest degree attained, 1978. *(Original artwork based on data provided by ANA and NLN.)*

sented the development of large-scale federal initiatives in nursing education at both preparatory and advanced levels. (Earlier federal programs were limited to the support of public health nursing and the establishment of the Cadet Nurses Corps under the exigencies of the Second World War.) By 1970, the *Progress Report on Nurse Training* [26] could summarize a number of accomplishments that the report attributed in large part to the infusion of federal support. These included:

1   An increase in both the quality and quantity of programs for nursing education.
2   A shift in student enrollment from non-collegiate to collegiate preparatory programs.
3   Awards in excess of $15 million to improve the quality of instruction in nursing programs.
4   Provision of more than 30,000 traineeships, together with more than 100,000 low-interest loans and educational opportunity grants to needy students.

Although some of the points may be arguable—for example, an increase in admissions to the nursing preparatory programs might have occurred over these years even in the absence of federal funding—the general conclusions seem to be fairly limited and reasonable.

As a result of the *Progress Report* and an earlier *Program Review Report* [27], the Nurse Training Act of 1971 expanded the already established programs and added the general category of capitation funds: direct payments to schools for each student enrolled provided the total enrollment was increased by a designated percentage each year [28]. As a consequence of these expanded sources of aid, one estimate indicated that in 1972 the federal government was supplying as much as

10 percent of all funding for nursing education programs [29]. In turn, the very provision of these funds seemed to spark greater attention from state and local government to the needs of nursing education and the support of its institutions. This was facilitated, moreover, by the altered patterns emerging within the preparatory programs. More than 80 percent of the hospital training programs were in private institutions; more than 80 percent of the associate degree programs were in public institutions. As the former declined and the latter expanded, the base of tax support and governmental funding shifted significantly.

Nevertheless, by 1978 fiscal problems remained a high priority for educational administrators. The reasons are many and complex, but among the causes are these: the unpredictability of federal funds and decisions; the higher costs attached to clinical teaching generally; the long history of "deprivation" in nursing education prior to the Nurse Training Acts, which affects the level of need; and the more recent period of inflation plus recession, which has increased the costs of operation and, simultaneously, put pressure on both public and private institutions to reduce, postpone, or eliminate expenditures that otherwise might have gone into program improvements and enlargement.

The infusion of federal, state, and private dollars for the improvement of teaching facilities is underscored by the decrease in its priority ranking as a problem in 1978. This decrease must also be recognized, however, as a partial consequence of the internal changes taking place in numbers and kinds of preparatory programs: those that were the weakest on several counts, including facilities and structures, have largely disappeared. Thus, in some respects, the reordering of needs for help with "bricks and mortar" is an artifact of external conditions rather than the consequence of systematic programs for planning, support, and construction. Or, put another way, it may be the emergence of an even more pressing problem.

In 1968, the deans and directors of preparatory programs ranked the implementation of change as a very distant fourth priority. In 1978, that problem was the third highest priority in the Hagopian survey and was even more pronounced in the responses to our staff survey of a stratified sample of all three general forms of preparatory programs. The pace of activity both within and without the profession demanded change and innovation, and the heads of programs were quick to perceive the pressures on them to formulate responses. Among the greatest needs they saw were for the determination of real differences between associate and baccalaureate programs, the articulation of these programs and their institutions, general planning for the future of American nursing education, the development of new leaders and changed styles of leadership, and the creation of new relationships between educators and nursing service personnel, particularly in terms of increasing the involvement of faculty members in clinical practice and ongoing patient care.

Many of these high-priority concerns, particularly those of articulation and unification (the recombination of nursing education and service), were hardly items for discussion in 1968. A decade later, they represented both challenge and promise —fraught with real perils in transition and enactment.

Innovation and change undoubtedly also are reflected in the citation of need for curricular development by the heads of programs. Although its priority ranking was unchanged between 1968 and 1978, the difference in frequency of mention was significant and pronounced. The emergence of the expanded role of the nurse in primary care, the need for better conceptual frameworks for the care of wellness and illness, the pressures for specialized clinical practitioners in an ever increasing number of fields, and the emphasis on graduate and continuing education as a natural progression of learning and experiential development all combined to call for a reexamination of everything that is traditional in the education of American nurses.

It is in the light of these pressures and conditions, for example, that the Nursing Curriculum Project of the Southern Regional Education Board (SREB) felt compelled to go back to the very basics of educational planning through a process that identified:

1   The kinds of workers needed and the competencies that were required for patient care and delivery
2   A taxonomy of competencies and strategies required for each level of practice
3   A body of knowledge related to the educational development of the identified competencies
4   A recommended plan for implementation

This reformulation of nursing education represents a vastly different approach to problem identification and solution than the more typical patchwork attempts that individuals or even institutions might instigate in the face of a felt need or problem [30]. It is conceptually akin to the process of zero-base budgeting, in which one starts with a tabula rasa and constructs a whole new system based on fresh assumptions, studied tables of needs and priorities, and a reexamination of the entire corpus of knowledge and information and skill required in the performance of the determined behaviors.

Overall, although the problems facing preparatory institutions look much the same when they are listed and catalogued, below the surface there is greater complexity and less uniformity than appeared to be the case over a decade ago. Our survey data indicated that problems are for the most part more pressing—and more difficult to solve—but, at the same time, there is a healthy recognition that diverse approaches are required and acceptable and that an enlightened heterodoxy is preferable to dogmatic approaches that too often failed in the past to reach effective and efficient resolutions.

It would not be complete to leave the discussion concerning Table 5–3 without providing some additional information elicited from our staff survey of diploma, associate degree, and baccalaureate institutions. In addition to our inquiries concerning the greatest needs and the most significant trends that these deans and directors perceived as impacting on their programs, we attempted to assess the potency of these problems in terms of the felt difficulty of solution. This query sought to order the problems of nursing education in terms of the greatest difficulties anticipated in effecting their resolution. This alternative view of the world of institutional challenges is displayed in Table 5–4.

Table 5-4   Tabulation of "Most Difficult Problems to Solve" in Nursing
Education as Perceived by Deans and Directors of Diploma, Associate,
and Baccalaureate Programs, 1978

Problem	Relative weighted value
1. Financial problems	61
2. Professional leadership, direction, and cohesion	60
3. More qualified faculty	36
4. Career mobility and articulation	34
5. Production of more competent graduates	33
6. Role confusion and changes	29
7. Conflict between nursing education and service	28
8. Determination of appropriate competency levels	27
9. Adequate clinical facilities	21

The categorization of problems ranked by potency or difficulty of solution
provides a useful long-term view of the needs of the entire profession. There are real
needs for change and curriculum development, but the abiding nature of financial
needs and shortcomings obviously must be addressed and solutions found. Similarly,
the perceived lack of cohesion and direction mentioned in response to an open-ended
query argues for the need to develop a unified House of Nursing as a prerequisite
to the assault on many more specific concerns. If one wished to develop an agenda
for professionalization, the information in Table 5–4 provides priorities for one to
ponder. In combination with Table 5–3, the problems can be arranged into short-,
mid-, and long-term needs that are challenging enough for any emerging profession.

In examining the specific recommendations made by the National Commission
for the Study of Nursing and Nursing Education in 1970 for the relief of the
problems impinging on preparatory programs, those recommendations that dealt
with the increase of federal and state outlays for faculty development and facilities
enhancement were realized at least in part, and precedents have been set for future
programming. In the case of two specific proposals aimed at alleviating these kinds
of problems, the outcomes are more ambiguous and less encouraging.

In 1970, the Commission pointed out that, in the decade ending in 1966, the
average number of students per school had climbed from 103 to 114. This information indicated that there were a large number of preparatory institutions that admitted very small numbers of students, with consequent problems in terms of per capita
cost, faculty acquisition, and curricular quality. We proposed that small programs
be terminated and that any institution that consistently admitted less than 25 students should seriously address the matter of its continuance. In 1978, the average
number of students per institution had climbed to approximately 185, due in part
to the termination of many small hospital training programs. There remain, however, a number of schools with low admissions, and in light of the recurrent problems
of finances, faculty, and facilities, it would seem that state master planning committees and other groups charged with the concerns of overall direction of nursing
education should scrutinize those programs that today admit less than 50 students

on a consistent basis—and in some areas even this figure may be too conservative for effective utilization of scarce resources.

A second Commission proposal dealt with the regional institution of faculty sharing and joint appointment, as well as aggressive programming for faculty development. The deans and directors report little activity in the areas of interinstitutional sharing of faculty, but indicate a considerable growth in such areas as programs for individual faculty development opportunities. Both the W. K. Kellogg Foundation and the Robert Wood Johnson Foundation have supported activities and programs designed to enhance the clinical skills of nurse faculty members, and the nursing group within the Southern Regional Education Board has mounted an interstate and panregional approach to faculty development programming. Current needs would seem, however, to far outstrip the available resources, and a reexamination of the concept of faculty sharing and interinstitutional academic appointments might prove to be extremely worthwhile for the next several years.

ACCREDITATION OF EDUCATIONAL INSTITUTIONS

In its *Abstract for Action,* the National Commission recognized that nursing had been almost singular among the health care professions in having its institutional accreditation policies and practices under the control of an organization, the National League for Nursing, which inherently provided for nonnurse membership, leadership, and policymaking activities. Thus, nursing was better positioned than most other health care professions to affirm that responsibility of accreditation which is, "To meet fully its obligations both to its members and society . . . that consideration will be given in their actions and policies to the public interest" [31].

There was, however, in 1970 an increasing concern about both the multiplicity of accrediting procedures across the health care professions and the validity of public representation on most of these bodies. Moreover, every accrediting agency has a tendency to develop an idealized model of an exemplary educational program and to have a resultant reluctance to accept innovative patterns and procedures that vary from the normative characteristics of the accepted and valued approach.

For all these reasons, the Commission proposed that a national committee be jointly established by the NLN and ANA to study and recommend future accrediting procedures that would ensure that actions and policies were in interest of the public as well as that of members and that provision be made for both changing institutional patterns and the concurrent activities taking place among other health professions.

In 1974, the House of Delegates of the ANA voted to "examine the feasibility of basic and graduate accreditation by the ANA" and gave immediate impetus to the concept of an interorganizational study. Both the National League for Nursing and the American Association of Colleges of Nursing were invited to participate in two conferences designed to discuss the concerns of accreditation. Out of these meetings came the proposal to enlarge the purview of a formal study commission to include the entire credentialing process—including not only accreditation, but licensure, certification, academic degrees, and all other forms of professional documentation.

Eventually, in 1976, the American Nurses' Association determined to sponsor the study on its own, but with the understanding that three types of cooperating agencies would be involved throughout the investigation. These were organizations with nurse members, structural units of health-related organizations whose members are nurses, and organizations whose major concerns relate to nursing. Over time, some 70 agencies and organizations were consulted with and involved in the credentialing study.

Explicit in the recommendation of the National Commission was that the membership of the study group include some numbers of nonnurses. In August of 1976, fifteen members were appointed: ten nurses and five others. The NLN officially decline to cosponsor the study, but members and staff cooperated with the committee and its staff. Although the membership of the committee was both distinguished and broadly representative, it is important to point out that four groups were not included which had been specifically suggested in *An Abstract for Action.* These were the regional accrediting associations, higher education associations, the office of the U.S. Commissioner of Education, and the National Commission on Accrediting. It was the feeling of the National Commission for the Study of Nursing and Nursing Education that these groups not only could contribute to the quality of any study, but also would be essential to the implementation of any significant changes pursuant to the findings and recommendations of the investigation. Time will be the best judge and perhaps the concerns of 1970 were overdrawn.

In 1979, the Report of the Committee for the Study of Credentialing in Nursing was released. The wide-ranging discussions touched upon basic definitions and principles as well as critical issues and recommendations. In particular, the committee addressed the control of credentialing, its costs, the assurance of competence, and the accountability of the profession and its credentialing agencies—as well as state and federal units that become involved in such processes [32].

In its key formulation of a basic position on control of credentialing, the committee stated:

1   It is appropriate for state agencies to license individuals for practice;

2   It is appropriate for the profession, with broad consultation, to credential individuals for entry into professional and specialty practice and to credential institutions offering educational programs for entry into practice and for entry into specialty practice, as well as to credential institutions providing organized nursing services.

3   It is appropriate for the federal government to determine that agencies and individuals eligible for funding and reimbursement are credentialed according to the roles defined above.

These propositions would require a basic reformulation of the relationships among the profession, public agencies, and the service organizations that hire and utilize nurses. Even in the case of the educational institutions, the expanded view of accreditation as a subset of the greater process of credentialing would generate new challenges and interactions. In this respect, a highly significant definition and position is advanced in the section on the *Definitions of Nursing:*

> 1 Nursing practices should be defined by the professional society. [This is a generic term referring to what is currently the ANA.]*

The full import of this simple statement cannot be underestimated. At present, the credentialing of entry into practice is governed by state boards of nursing with or without the definitions of the professional society. Entry into specialized practice is often monitored by specialty practice groups outside the ANA and is occasionally regulated by specific powers of state boards of nursing. Institutional accrediting of educational programs at various levels is handled by the NLN, which is, by definition, not a professional society, and certainly not the ANA. Moreover, hospitals and other care agencies have long been involved in some aspects of credentialing, as have medical societies and specialty practice groups. So, while saying that nursing practice should be defined by the professional society for purposes of credentialing, the committee essentially calls for a fundamental and far-reaching turn of events.

The report of the Committee for the Study of Credentialing in Nursing deserves thoughtful consideration and response. In detailing the impact of the one proposition for professional determination and definition of nursing, for example, it revealed one of the basic flaws not only of credentialing in nursing, but also of accreditation in many of the emergent health care bodies. So many diverse agencies, organizations, and interest groups are involved in these activities which have little commonality of purpose, less agreement on levels and scope of practice, and, all too frequently, an exaggerated sense of territoriality that our present approach to the entire business is that of a nonsystem. Any constructive suggestions merit examination, and the committee in presenting its report initiated the process of discussion and review, critique and commentary.

As the agency for carrying out the diverse activities of credentialing individuals and institutions, the committee recommended the creation of a free-standing Nursing Credentialing Center that could enlist the cooperation and support of all the organizations and agencies that would feel the impact of the changed procedures and regulations. As an interim step, the committee further called for the establishment of a Task Force broadly representative of nursing and the public. This body would serve as the catalyst and the energizer to develop support for the basic concept of the credentialing center and to initiate the operational planning and cost analyses that would be necessary to the start-up of such an organization.

The data gathering and the problem identification activities of the committee staff have gone a long way toward highlighting the concerns that the National Commission expressed in 1970; the resultant approaches and recommendations are far more wide-ranging than anticipated in *An Abstract for Action.* It is now up to

---

*Since the ANA funded the credentialing study, it is understandable that the ANA is accepted as the *professional society* in this definition. Many nurses and nursing organizations would demur.

the nursing organizations to decide on the fundamental issues raised by the committee and the future directions limned out by that body.

CURRICULAR NEEDS AND ARTICULATION

One of the most troublesome areas in all nursing education in 1968 was curriculum development and articulation. Two particular shortcomings were identified by the educational advisory panel to the Commission: the first was a lack of interinstitutional planning among the various kinds of preparatory programs to facilitate upward career mobility; the second was a lack of differentiation among the objectives of the then existent programs to cover the wide variety of needs that patient care demanded.

These two conditions, viewed together, represented a strange paradox in educational planning. The lack of a curricular ladder was due in large part to the fact that the various preparatory institutions for nursing education often worked in splendid isolation. Baccalaureate and higher degree programs, for example, seldom met or planned with their counterparts from diploma or associate degree programs. Tacit acceptance was given to the assertion that 2-year programs were technical and terminal and that transfer would be most difficult, if not impossible, into a baccalaureate program. At the same time, however *all* of the various programs displayed a pronounced proclivity for centering their curricula around the service need areas of the hospital setting. Courses, clinical training, and licensure examinations all reflected the heavy emphasis on preparing nurses for the acute care setting. So deeply imbued was this approach that many nurse educators saw this not as a specialization, but rather as a general, undifferentiated entry into practice. Considerable apprehension was displayed particularly by those who saw the generic baccalaureate program as the single best way to prepare all nurses for their professional roles, since their assumptions were challenged by the demand for both vertical and horizontal reconstruction. It is to the credit of nursing that both institutions and individuals have taken up the challenge to reconsider their entire educational curriculum.

Vertical Reconstruction

When *An Abstract for Action* proposed, in 1970, that there be planned curricular articulation between 2- and 4-year programs such that the transfer of graduates from the lower-division programs would be facilitated, the concept was not without precedent although it struck many nurse educators as a revolutionary practice. Gwynedd-Mercy College had established an associate degree program in nursing in 1959 and an upper-division baccalaureate program in 1968. Graduates of diploma programs, transfer graduates from other associate degree programs, and Gwynedd-Mercy's own 2-year nurses alike completed the baccalaureate degree with a minimum of difficulty in admissions and placement [33]. In the same time period, Chioni and others had developed the experimental baccalaureate program at the University of Wisconsin, which ran through 4 years and which provided access for R.N.s on an individual assessment basis [34]. Dustan and her colleagues at Iowa also had developed a curricular plan to establish an interrelated lower- and upper-division sequence leading to the associate degree followed by the baccalaureate degree in nursing [35].

The National Commission felt, however, that in order to realize the promise of these pioneering efforts there had to be regional and interstitutional planning and demonstration projects to display the practicality and generalizability of the concept. The Southern Regional Education Board Nursing Curriculum Project and the Orange County/Long Beach Corsortium Project became particular tests of the value of vertical reconstruction of the nursing curriculum.

From 1972 through 1975, the SREB Nursing Curriculum Project sought to develop a professional consensus on the levels of competency required of nurses at different stages of preparation and experience. It grouped role expectations into three general categories: functional behaviors, human or interpersonal competencies, and conceptual formulations. Out of an extensive examination of both traditional and emergent care requirements, the SREB seminar participants then prepared a taxonomy of anticipated abilities related to the academic level of the nurse practitioner. One example, from the area of conceptual formulations, is displayed in Figure 5–6. Note that the recognition and use of information related to patient condition and care is a *universal* curricular concern for the most part, whereas the manipulation and analysis of information at higher levels of conceptual processing become *distinctive* or *differentiating* curricular concerns [36]. Coupled with the taxonomies of functional and interpersonal competence, the SREB model provides a systematic view of appropriate discrimination in curriculum planning at each collegiate academic level.

The Orange County/Long Beach Consortium for Nursing Education developed an interinstitutional model for systematic articulation of nursing education which could conceivably develop behavioral competencies from the nurse aide level on through the clinical/research doctorate. Emphasis was placed on the formulation of specific behaviors for each level so that the exit competencies at any given level would become the entrance requirements and expectations for the next higher level [37]. A schematic outline of the overall schema is displayed in Figure 5–7, and an organizational chart of the institutional relationships is shown in Figure 5–8. The resemblance of Figure 5–8 to the general proposal of the National Commission for the Study of Nursing and Nursing Education as presented in Figure 5–1 is, of course, a deliberate effort to implement that recommendation and develop the tactical skills and resources necessary to make the idea operational.

To illustrate the differentiation in competencies that were described in behavioral terms for each level, graduates of the consortium associate degree programs were expected to

1 Transfer knowledge from biological and behavioral sciences to nursing situations

2 Make nursing judgments and establish priorities in directing and evaluating the care of individual patients and groups of patients

	ADN	BSN	MSN	DSN
CONCEPTUAL COMPETENCIES: GENERAL				
Recognizes Information				
Description of events	▬	▬	▬	▬
Generalizations	▬	▬	▬	▬
Facts	▬	▬	▬	▬
Laws-principles-concepts	▬	▬	▬	▬
Theories-models	▬	▬	▬	▬
Uses Information				
Understands (compares, para-phrases, translates, interprets) information concerning:				
descriptions of events and situations	▬	▬	▬	▬
generalizations	▬	▬	▬	▬
facts	▬	▬	▬	▬
laws-principles-concepts	▬	▬	▬	▬
theories-models		▬	▬	▬
Manipulates Information				
Employs problem-solving methods:				
using several cues	▬	▬	▬	▬
using many more cues		▬	▬	▬
using complex cues			▬	▬
emphasizing intersystem conceptualizations				▬
Selects data to be collected:				
traditional and routine	▬	▬	▬	▬
above and beyond routine		▬	▬	▬
goes beyond information readily available			▬	▬
Uses data selected:				
as prescribed	▬	▬	▬	▬
above and beyond prescription		▬	▬	▬
Forms ideas and hypotheses concerning data	▬	▬	▬	▬
Tests fit of data to event or situation:				
simple tests and constructs		▬	▬	▬
tests many more alternatives and constructs			▬	▬
complex tests and constructs				▬
Evaluates feedback data				

Figure 5–6   Excerpt from a taxonomy for conceptual competencies developed for the SREB nursing curriculum project. *(From the SREB nursing curriculum project. Used with permission.)*

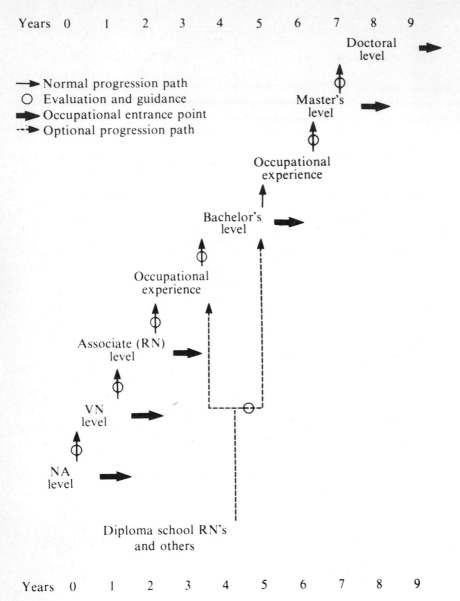

Figure 5–7   Schematic diagram of the articulated model for nursing education of the Orange County/Long Beach Consortium.

   3   Identify major manifestations of common health problems at varying patient age levels and know the expected results of medical treatment
   4   Interpret physician's orders and translate these into nursing action

In contrast to these A.D.N.-exit, B.S.N.-entrance behaviors, the B.S.N. graduate of the consortium programs would be expected to

1   Focus on care of clients in health care facilities where nursing roles are numerous and diffuse

2   Demonstrate leadership ability as a member of the health team

3   Assume primary care functions such as history taking, physical assessment, psychosocial assessment, diagnosis, triage, treatment and/or referral, and follow-up

4   Assume a facilitative role in teaching and guiding co-workers in the provision of client care

Each of these general statements would be amplified by specific behavior explications that would, in sum, demonstrate to the instructor that the competency was mastered

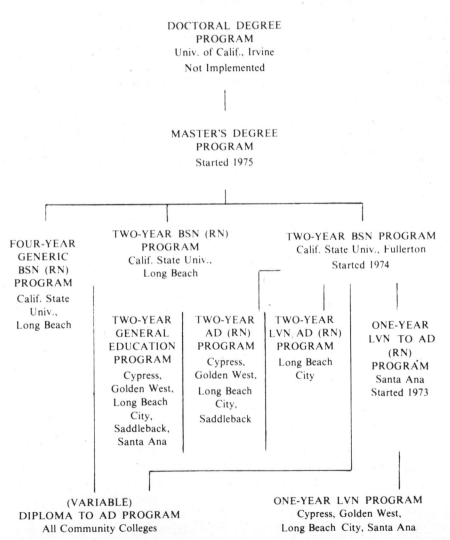

Figure 5–8   Organizational relationships of the Orange County/Long Beach Consortia institutions.

by the learner. The total of the terminal behaviors of the baccalaureate nurse, then, became the entrance competencies for the master's degree programs within the consortium.

An increasing number of institutions have begun to develop curricular plans based on the two-plus-two or lower-upper division concept. In our survey of baccalaureate programs in nursing in 1978, approximately 36 percent of the responding institutions indicated that there was some form of special approach taken toward the transfer of associate degree graduates. Approximately 57 percent of the respondents indicated that no special provision existed for articulation of these students at the current time. No less than 61 percent of all the baccalaureate programs surveyed, however, were involved in some form of institutional planning for the articulation of the curriculum between the separate preparatory levels, so prospects for the future are hopeful if not optimistic. Still further encouragement is provided by the emergence of a number of baccalaureate programs designed strictly as upper-division institutions for the baccalaureate education of associate degree graduates. All in all, considerable progress has taken place in terms of the vertical reconstruction of the nursing curriculum.

Horizontal Reconstruction

From its inception, the National Commission emphasized that its first objective was the improvement of health care through the refinement of nursing practice, education, and careers. Very early in the investigation, however, it became obvious that the traditional role of the nurse in acute illness settings, important as it was and is, was too exclusive a concern in curricular formation. Based on extensive site visits and interviews, it was clear in 1968 that dramatic changes had taken place in three important dimensions that, taken together, tended to define the role expectations for nursing practice. Nurses were working across a broad continuum of client needs, from well patients through the midly unwell to the acutely ill. Care settings were similarly becoming more differentiated, ranging from the client's home through the short-term facility to the long-term institution. At the same time, nurses not only were providing direct care, but also were required to do more assessment and diagnosis, as well as more health teaching and evaluation, than ever before.

Significantly, it was the experiential world of practice that was shaping these new patterns and roles. As Prock later observed, "Role innovation in nursing either in public health or in institutional nursing has not come from the faculties in schools of nursing . . . the impetus for creating and using these new roles in nursing has come from the fields of practice" [38]. It was essential, however, that educational courses and curricula be reorganized and updated in terms of the actuality of care demands.

Lest the reaction to the changing role expectations for nursing result in an extreme swing into narrow specialization at too early a point in preparatory programs, the National Commission called for the development of concentrations in episodic or distributive practice to be built on a general core of nursing knowledge, skills, and theory. It was conceivable that "concentrations" rather than "specializations" could be accommodated within both associate degree and baccalaureate competencies, with a higher degree of specialty practice perhaps being emphasized in the upper-division matrix.

If anything, the initial response of conservative nurse educators to this proposal was more hostile than that to vertical reconstruction. Some, unaware that the practice roles for clinical nursing had changed so dramatically, simply opposed any change in the status quo. Others sincerely felt that so-called generic programs for nursing preparation were generalizable to all beginning nursing requirements—steadfastly overlooking the medical/hospital service implications that undergirded almost every aspect of the curriculum. A few came close to espousing a conspiracy theory that viewed the proposal for reconstruction as a ploy to subdivide nursing into a host of technical skill areas with no catholic concerns and commitments.

Fortunately, reflection and consideration replaced resentment and conjecture. The SREB Nursing Curriculum Project noted, for example, that "nursing practice will include a multitude of workers who will differ in their use of nursing behaviors varying with the setting in which services are given, the nature of control concerning the decision-making process within that setting, and the nature of the client to be served" [39]. Having thus affirmed the observations and schema of the National Commission staff, the project then proposed that "entry-level practice will be distinct for graduates of educational programs at different levels . . . and will require more conceptual and human competencies from graduates of upper-division programs" [40].

In fact, the SREB formulations actually went far beyond the National Commission's proposals for restructuring the horizontal dimensions of the nursing curriculum. Whereas *An Abstract for Action* called for differentiated clinical concentrations at the associate and baccalaureate levels, the SREB proposal examined the need for concentrations in research, administration, organization, and education as well as clinical specialization and formulated a conceptual scheme by relating this information about concentrations to the board's proposed changes in the vertical dimension of curricular articulation. The board's proposal for the comprehensive curriculum for future American nursing is presented in Figure 5–9.

This differentiation of levels and specialties gives some substantive meaning to the terms *vertical* and *horizontal* mobility. It also provides a comprehensive challenge to curriculum developers, who must bridge the gap between preparation and practice in such ways that never again will role innovation in nursing be seen as being unrelated to the programs of preparatory institutions.

In order to determine the extent to which preparatory programs have moved toward horizontal curricular reconstruction, our survey of educational institutions included two questions:

1 Does your institution offer clinical concentrations in episodic or distributive care?
2 Does your institution offer clinical concentrations based on a conceptual scheme other than episodic/distributive care?

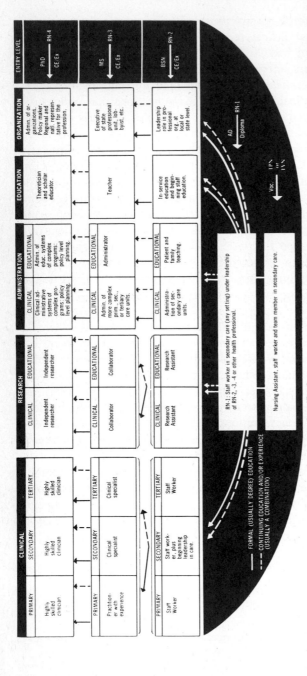

Figure 5–9 Proposed future curricular tracks for nursing specialist levels as formulated by the SREB nursing curriculum project. *(From American Journal of Nursing and SREB nursing curriculum project. Used with permission.)*

Table 5-5   Institutions Providing Clinical Concentrations Based on Episodic/Distributive Care Formulations

Type of institution	Yes		No		No response	
	Number	Percent	Number	Percent	Number	Percent
Baccalaureate	32	46	31	45	6	7
Associate degree	22	26	58	69	4	5
Diploma	22	44	26	52	2	4
Total	76	37	115	57	12	6

The results are displayed in Tables 5–5 and 5–6. Overall, more than one out of three of the respondents had revised their curricula to offer clinical concentrations in episodic or distributive care. Baccalaureate institutions were highest, with 46 percent compliance; associate degree programs were lowest, with 26 percent. Among institutions that had not adopted the particular conceptual formation proposed by the National Commission, there was still considerable movement toward alternative forms of clinical concentrations at the preparatory level. Of these respondents, 29 percent overall had elective concentrations while a few indicated that they were assessing the possibility of instituting such curricular alternatives in the near future.

In sum, two out of every three preparatory institutions responding to our survey (67 percent) have instituted some form of clinical concentration in the curriculum. Of those that have done so, more than half (56 percent) have used the episodic/distributive concept as the guideline for curriculum planning. Perhaps the most encouraging result of the survey is that a total of 78 percent of all the responding baccalaureate institutions have adopted some form of clinical concentration arrangement designed to achieve the purposes envisaged in the recommendations of the National Commission for the reorganization of the horizontal dimension of the nursing preparatory curriculum.

There are, of course, many problems yet to be resolved in terms of the nursing curriculum. By our survey, it would appear that approximately 50 percent of the associate degree programs have provided for elective concentrations—meaning that half of these instutional curricula are still essentially aimed at episodic, acute nursing practice only. Greater refinement is necessary. It will be necessary for the majority of nurse graduates to assume clinical positions and responsibilities within the hospital and acute care settings of the American health care delivery system for a long

Table 5-6   Institutions Providing Clinical Concentrations Based on Conceptual Schema Other than Episodic/Distributive

Type of institution	Yes		No		No response	
	Number	Percent	Number	Percent	Number	Percent
Baccalaureate	22	32	39	57	8	11
Associate degree	20	24	56	67	8	9
Diploma	17	34	26	52	7	14
Total	59	29	121	60	8	9

period to come, but the need for distributive nursing practice is increasing in significant fashion. The combination of curricular unfreezing and state master planning committees may go a long way toward ensuring that we are able to produce the correct mixture of varied kinds of nurse professionals to undertake the dictates of patient care.

In 1970, the National Commission added a caveat to its recommendations for horizontal reformulation of nursing curricula. It suggested that many nursing programs preferred the utilization of nursing faculty alone in developing specialized programs for nursing education and administration. In the light of the SREB formulations for additional programs in organization and research, this tendency may become more pronounced. It is no criticism of the profession to remind nursing that it may profitably seek the assistance of other disciplines and professions in the development of advanced specialized skills in an area such as administration. The highest priority of the nursing profession is to produce competent clinicians capable of providing care across the universe of patient needs, care settings, and appropriate functional interventions. Beyond this, nursing, as any other discipline or profession, should be chary of investing time, resources, and human capital in doing what others can provide as a matter of course in their own fields of competence. To argue for nursing's independence is not to propose professional insularity.

If this concern seems overdrawn, let us speak simply to the point. In the site interviews and surveys of nursing students conducted for the purposes of this longitudinal follow-up to *An Abstract for Action,* it is still apparent that many faculty members are perceived—rightly or wongly—as being aloof from and unconcerned with the clinical roles and responsibilities of the profession. In a challenging and worthy curriculum, it is essential that students encounter faculty with rich and varied background, but the first essential of excellence in a clinical profession is, and of a right ought to be, the portrayal of a role model in patient care. Faculty members should be excellent nurses. Over and above this, they may be historians, lawyers, sociologists, and zoologists. But when they shun responsibility for and participation in clinical patient care, then they have ceased to be professional nurses in the true sense of the term. It is this concern that prompts the reiteration of the basic Commission tenet: The true study of nurses is nursing, in its full dimensions, across the broad range of patient needs, and in the widest possible settings.

Tremendous progress has been made in the development of a reconstructed horizontal dimension to the nursing curriculum. In 1968, the number of nursing programs with varied and in-depth clinical electives could have been numbered by the fingers of a few hands. In 1978, the majority of baccalaureate programs and a significant number of associate degree programs began extensive curricular innovation. If the role of the National Commission was only to serve as an advocate and an irritant, the results would be satisfactory. The fact that so many preparatory institutions identify with the terminology and formulations of *An Abstract for Action* suggests a deeper causality. Credit and recognition, however, rightfully belong to those individual nurses and preparatory institutions that went beyond the limits of the status quo and reasserted the need for periodic reformulation of nursing education and related curricula.

GRADUATE STUDY AND FACULTY DEVELOPMENT

One of the harshest prices that was exacted by the problems of preparatory programs in nursing education was the consequent weakening of graduate studies and reduction in the number of individuals pursuing advanced work. A preliminary study in California prior to the beginning of the Orange County/Long Beach consortium, for example, showed that licensed vocational nurses often had to complete 6 years of study to fulfill the requirements of a baccalaureate degree in nursing! Such lack of program compatibility and consequent length of an undergraduate degree were poor harbingers for advanced or graduate education.

With the positioning of preparatory nursing programs within the collegiate mainstream of American education, however, the National Commission anticipated that there would be a dramatic growth in graduate admissions as a combination of increased demand and improved access. The results have, if anything, exceeded the most optimistic projections. In 1968, there were slightly more than 4000 master's degree students enrolled in some 65 colleges and universities. As indicated in Figure 5–10, there has been a threefold increase in the number of these students within the decade—an enrollment in excess of 12,000 in 1978. Relatedly, there are more than 115 institutions offering graduate programs at the present time. With increased admissions at more institutions, it seems quite probable that there will be 14,000 nurses enrolled in master's programs by 1982. As significant as these increases are, however, the need for advanced clinical practitioners for both nursing education and service still far exceeds the available supply.

The trends in doctoral education for nursing are similar. Up to 1968, there was an almost steady state in the number of institutions and enrollments. Approximately five doctoral programs enrolled 100 full-time students. By 1978, both of these numbers trebled and, in addition, an increasing number of nurses were completing doctoral programs in schools and departments other than nursing—in education,

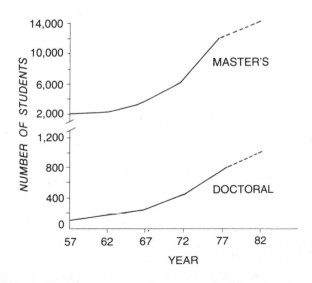

Figure 5–10 Trends in enrollment in master's and doctoral programs.

administration, and the various sciences. Altogether, however, there were only slightly more than 2000 nurses with earned doctorates in the entire country.

When one considers the need for administrative leadership, educational direction, and clinical research into improved patient care, then the deficits in advanced nursing education become painfully clear. Disciplines and professions that customarily view the earned doctorate as the entry level for practice simply cannot comprehend the difficulties encountered by a clinical group in which one-tenth of one percent of the individual members have been prepared at the doctoral level. Using the conservative analyses of the UCLA Health Manpower Project, for example, one would estimate that current needs of nursing would require 20,000 nurses trained at the doctoral level simply to meet the minimal responsibilities for education and service [41]. Nursing currently "enjoys" one-tenth of that number, but it carries responsibility for the direction of clinical nursing services in thousands of hospitals, nursing homes, and varied health facilities and, at the same time, is conducting preparatory and advanced educational activities through more than 1500 institutional programs.

There is no quick or easy solution to this dilemma. Current doctoral programs in nursing face problems in acquiring a "critical mass" of qualified faculty, so that adding more programs would only compound the difficulties of the present. Moreover, the tangible nature of unfilled, budgeted positions for doctorally prepared nurses at the deanship or clinical directorship level tends to compel people into administrative fields and away from both practice and research—although the latter are emphasized in most nursing doctoral programs. One essentially ends up running faster and faster just to remain in place. Scarce resources coupled with almost unlimited needs can provide great opportunity, but when the gulf between resource and need is as vast as in American nursing, the situation is fraught with elements of frustration, failure, and futility.

The frequency of turnover in leadership positions, the competition for doctorally prepared individuals, and the pressure on everyone to excel in multiple fields simultaneously are very real signs and symptoms of illness. The cure can be realized only by the development, over time, of an adequate supply of doctorally prepared nurses, certainly no less than the 20,000 called for in the assessment of current needs. Relief, however, could be realized by a self-imposed moratorium on creating new graduate programs, by a commitment to offer (and accept) jobs that are truly related to one's preparation and experience, and by a willingness to establish professional priorities in such ways that practice and research are encouraged and are seen as essential activities for doctorally prepared nurses.

For the remainder of this century, graduate study and faculty development will continue to be precarious. The deficits in current preparation beyond the baccalaureate level will not be made up quickly or easily. Moreover, the growing emphasis on revitalizing the clinical skills of nursing faculty at all levels will add a challenging dimension to in-service program planning. In the SREB Nursing Curriculum project alone, there are four demonstration sites devoted to the upgrading of clinical skills among faculty members. Any expansion of the so-called unification model for teaching and practice will geometrically increase the need for clinical retraining and instruction. The impact will be both to upgrade the quality of all nursing education and to enhance the overall image of the profession, but the effort required will be enormous.

It should be noted that nursing, in 1968, showed a very promising interest in the application of new instructional approaches and technology to the education of all students, undergraduate and graduate, and that the resultant materials and methods were beginning to be utilized in continuing and in-service education. In surveys, discussions, and interviews in 1978, the Commission found that innovative education seemed to be an even more active field of endeavor, with self-instructional laboratories, simulators, and individualized teaching materials expanding their impact. In the face of the scarcity of human resources, the innovative use of technology is a singularly helpful addition to the teaching-learning process and merits continued development and enlargement.

INSTITUTIONAL ADMISSION AND RETENTION

A decade ago, the National Commission for the Study of Nursing and Nursing Education examined and commented on three aspects of institutional admission and retention. The most problematic issue dealt with the freedom of admission into any nursing program upon completion of a lower level of preparation. A second concern had to do with the recruitment and admission of minority groups into educational programs. The third had to do with the retention of all students in all programs in order to achieve the highest possible levels of successful completion. The Commission recommended increased efforts toward the accomplishment of all three goals. It must be stressed, in all this, that nursing as a profession had pioneered many of the attempts to attract minority students and had demonstrated a constructive concern over retention efforts and results. As a result, much of what the Commission proposed was the encouragement of activities already under way and the systematic expansion of programs over time.

Our survey in 1978 indicated that over half of our sample of preparatory institutions had done formal planning for educational articulation and admissions from lower programs and just over half (51 percent) had developed a systematic plan for facilitating such arrangements. Within the subsets of the sample, there were impressive efforts to address particular admission needs for the sake of career mobility. For example, 76 percent of the surveyed junior and community colleges had planned programs to help licensed practical nurses complete the requirements for the R.N. Likewise, 56 percent of the hospital programs had L.P.N. to R.N. routes to facilitate upward mobility. One out of every three associate degree programs had planned arrangements for aides and other health workers below the L.P.N. level to complete L.P.N. and/or R.N. requirements. Among baccalaureate institutions, 36 percent reported having specialized programs for A.D.N. students seeking to complete the B.S.N. Although much remains to be done, the widespread nature of the positive response to date is most encouraging.

In terms of admitting minority students, the effort has been commendable. Of the baccalaureate institutions surveyed, 59 percent had established specific programs for the attraction and admission of minorities; among hospital schools and associate degree programs this percentage dropped to approximately 43 percent. The comments accompanying the survey replies, however, shed further insight into the current state of these efforts. One hundred percent of the responding institutions indicated an awareness of and concern for minority admissions, but 51 percent of the entire sample indicated that they enjoyed large numbers of applications from a wide variety of minority groups such that they did not require a specific program of recruitment or admission.

With regard to problems of retention and withdrawal, there is little indication that these should be a concern. In a philosophic sense, any loss between admission and graduation might be regrettable. On the other hand, so many decisions to enter nursing are made at an early age, with almost no personal experience of the rigors and the requirements for professional entry behavior, that a much higher loss could be anticipated than is actually experienced. Net retention rates for all preparatory nursing programs hover around 75 percent, with highest retention experienced by baccalaureate programs in private institutions and lowest retention found in public institutions offering baccalaureate programs. Attempts over the years to reduce withdrawals and other losses through screening tests and admissions batteries have proven largely fruitless; predictions based on such efforts have failed in terms of both validity and reliability. In short, the matter of retention seems to be operating within acceptable limits and should be viewed as having positive as well as negative properties. It is an area that deserves further investigation and experimentation, but in no way is it at a critical level of concern.

If there are two problems above the "threshold" limits in terms of admission and retention, they would be the perennial matter of sexual stereotyping in nursing and the lack of recruiting efforts among nontraditional but highly advantaged groups. Male students in nursing programs consistently run under 7 percent while the figure among practitioners is even more reduced. Nursing is seen as a female profession even more sharply than medicine is perceived to be a male occupation. Only time and cultural change can have more than minute impact on recruitment and admission of males into nursing.

An increasing number of preparatory programs in nursing have become aware of the advantages of recruiting graduates of arts and science programs into the profession. Despite the fact that most of these nursing programs offer a second baccalaureate rather than an entry-level master's degree, the admission of arts and science graduates is up and 20 percent of the baccalaureate programs responding to our 1978 survey indicated that they had specially planned programs for attracting and admitting such individuals to their institutions.

CONTINUING AND IN-SERVICE EDUCATION

In order to ensure that nurses would continue to maintain clinical expertise in the face of scientific and technological breakthroughs, and in an era of changing health care delivery systems, the National Commission for the Study of Nursing and Nursing Education proposed that the state master planning committees include continuing education, along with preparatory and graduate education, as a priority area demanding planning, coordination, and evaluation. Relatedly, the Commission called on health care facilities to upgrade and expand the in-service education of nurses in more specific training programs related to their job responsibilities and patient care requirements.

By 1978, no less than nine states had enacted laws requiring nurses to show evidence of continuing education in order to renew their licenses to practice. Another four states had passed permissive legislation enabling their boards of nursing to mandate such requirements. Many other states are studying the possibility of mandatory or voluntary systems for encouraging and supporting programs of continuing education for nurses.

In *An Abstract for Action,* the National Commission asserted the need to establish continued clinical competency as a requirement for relicensure, but separated that activity from the discussion of continuing education, believing that a system of voluntary involvement supported by professional organizations and associations might be superior to governmental intervention and the bureaucratic necessities that would accompany such an approach.

The thrust toward mandatory programming has been seen as a high-priority activity by many state nurses' associations, and the rapid advance of legislation in this area is a tribute to their effectiveness in marshaling support for the concept. Moreover, the American Nurses' Association, through its Council on Continuing Education in Nursing, has established standards for both the accreditation of continuing education programs and the accreditation of state nurses' associations and others as general providers and accreditation agents. The national prominence of the ANA has been a positive force in the development of common definitions and measures of quality, but there is still a wide variance among state requirements for relicensure, and the eventual impact on mobility and reciprocity among the states is difficult to judge at best.

Continuing education has become a large-scale enterprise. In those states that have mandated learning requirements for relicensure, problems have actually developed over how to provide the necessary courses and instructors to permit compliance. Several states have delayed the initiation date of the procedures in order to develop programs and facilities. Even in voluntary situations, there is growing interest in attending accredited continuing education programs, and an increasing number of entrepreneurs have joined traditional education and professional groups in offering continuing education and in-service training programs.

In the face of the growth and ferment over continuing education, two basic concerns still need to be addressed. The first of these is the relationship between continuing education and enhanced clinical skill and care. The basic purpose of requiring continuing education for health practitioners is to improve health care. One may accept uncritically the assertion that any good learning experience is capable of improving later clinical performance, but simple logic suggests that critical methods of evaluation should be invoked. Perusal of the catalogs and brochures for continuing education in nursing suggests a wide range in complexity, rigor, and clinical involvement. The clinical workshops of the American Association of Critical-Care Nurses or the continuing education programs of the Nurses' Association of the American College of Obstetricians and Gynecologists, for example, display a clear relationship between continuing education content and clinical application. On the other hand, an advertised course in Swahili may be relevant to a nurse in world health or missionary activities but is probably not the kind of continuing education experience envisaged by the individuals and organizations who fought so hard to make learning a lifelong professional commitment for nurses.

The second basic concern that should be monitored and objectively considered is the use of government agencies to enforce professional continuing education. The requirement that a nurse present 30 clock hours or a mixture of contact hours and self-study experiences can easily assume the posture of a lifeless standard. Any 30 hours of approved continuing education credit may be wholly unrelated to competent clinical development. It might be far better to have nurses pursuing continuing education programs for advanced certification or for expanded skills in physical assessment or primary care. An analogy might be drawn to professional education in New York State over the last decade. At the beginning of that period, one could obtain permanent certification in administration by acquiring 30 hours of graduate credit in that field after having been certified as a teacher. Later, the Board of Regents and the state education department required that each institution offering a program in educational administration draw up a "competency-based curriculum" of unspecified length or hours that would assure that the advanced training of individuals seeking permanent certification was related to behavioral goals and role requirements for such a position rather than being a mere collection of hours and courses. It is hoped that many of the states that have not mandated continuing education requirements for nurse relicensure can become experimental centers for alternative arrangements for assessing and enhancing continuing clinical growth among nurses without reducing the process to a simple numbers game.

One could, for example, accept continuing enrollment and progress in a clinical master's program as evidence for relicensure. Likewise, enrollment and progress in the certification program of the American Nurses' Association or of one of the specialty practice groups might be accepted. Participation in a regional program to promote primary care or physical assessment, as offered by some SREB institutions, could be viewed as a commitment to professional growth. Any or all of these programs intrinsically carry more overtones of clinical growth than does a standardized hour requirement. Herein lies a unique area for educational evaluation and research.

FINANCING OF THE RECOMMENDATIONS

In 1970, the National Commission noted that nursing education traditionally had been largely a matter of private and institutional financing, but there had appeared a marked trend toward higher levels of public support. In the face of evident needs for construction, institutional support, and student aid, the Commission proposed a minimum level of federal support for 1970 in the amount of $110 million and a desirable level of $125 million. The former figure was the same as that proposed for the Peace Corps, and neither amount looked large in the face of a budgetary outlay of $421 million simply for the removal of surplus commodities. In arriving at its figures and its distribution, however, the Commission observed that readjustments should be made in both amounts and categories over subsequent years.

Federal support for nursing was not a lengthy tradition in 1970. Nor were the amounts allocated to this profession very great by any standard of comparison. The Social Security Act of 1935 was the first instance of direct federal support of nursing education, and this was essentially an outgrowth of an effort to improve public health. Perhaps three thousand nurses received scholarships or awards for advanced training in public health. In 1943, the exigencies of the Second World War led to the passage of the Bolton Act and the establishment of the Cadet Nurse Corps to supply the increased numbers of nurses needed to meet the expanded military requirements. After the war emergency, this support was quietly terminated.

By 1956, the growing advances in medical research and hospital construction as well as the discussion of national health insurance led to a series of health manpower training acts designed to ensure that there were enough health workers to carry out the programs and policies formulated by the Congress and the Department of Health, Education, and Welfare (HEW). Included in those bills and amendments were traineeship grants for nurses seeking advanced education and some funding for nursing research. The unique aspects of nursing, however, as the largest of the health care professions and the most widely distributed across the entire realm of provider agencies, were singled out for support in the Nurse Training Act of 1964 [42]. This law provided funds for construction, teaching improvement, graduate traineeships, and low-interest student loans.

Later Nurse Training acts (NTA) and Health Manpower acts continued to widen the support for nursing education; the Nurse Training Act of 1971, for example, added the concept of capitation funding, sums of money provided to schools of nursing which increased their enrollment by designated percentages [43]. So rapidly had the federal government expanded its role in nursing education that it is estimated that, by 1972, 10 percent of all nursing school revenues were derived from federal programs. But these moneys also tended to have a generative effect upon other funds as well. The fact that the Congress and the several administrations emphasized the need for an adequate supply of nurses and committed strong support to enlarging the capabilities for educating increased numbers of practitioners persuaded many state and county governments to strengthen public support at more localized levels. Moreover, private foundations and philanthropies were encouraged to support new initiatives in education and clinical preparation.

Over these years of expansive federal programming, there began to emerge an increasing amount of political posturing in terms of the Manpower and Nurse Training acts. Congress frequently authorized more money than the administrations requested in their budgets—and more money than the Congress itself might later appropriate. To seasoned Washington observers, this was business as usual. To nursing schools and their administrators, it was an exasperating experience that severely affected long-range planning. When appropriations were much larger than budget requests, the Nixon administration experimented with the impoundment of funds, and when this practice was declared illegal, there was still pressure not to expend all the appropriated money. This was continued in the Ford administration, and in subsequent years actual funding has never reached the appropriation figures for programs established under the various Nurse Training acts. [44].

In November of 1978, President Carter vetoed the Nursing Training Act extension and timed the veto message so that it came after Congress had adjourned, thus ensuring there could be no quick override in reaction to his decision. On January 22, 1979, the President released his proposal for the 1980 federal budget, which included an 88 percent reduction in support for nursing and nursing education. Except for $14 million allocated to prepare advanced nurse practitioners, all support moneys have been eliminated from the Department of Health, Education, and Welfare. The reaction of the nursing profession was predictable and swift. The president of the American Nurses' Association declared that President Carter could not be "aware of the potential impact" of his action [45], and the *American Journal of Nursing* commented that "nursing education and the practice of nursing will suffer severely" and that the profession was facing its "most severe crises" in the wake of the administration's actions [46].

While congressional committees are pondering both the budgetary allocations and an executive request to rescind some $84 million appropriated for 1979, there is little doubt that tremendous pressure is being placed by the administration for the reduction and eventual elimination of all federal funding for nursing education.* Former Secretary of HEW Joseph Califano offered two explanations for this decision: (1) a shift in health manpower analyses from an assumption of an undersupply of nurses to one of surplus and (2) the general overextension of the federal budget and the need to cut support in many areas of health education and training [47].

Once again, the ambiguity of nursing's educational patterning has contributed to the confusion. Enough nurses are currently being graduated from preparatory programs to justify the first point made by Secretary Califano. What is not said, however, is that the retention rate in nursing is well below that of most other professions and, moreover, that we are still far short of establishing a system of articulated education that can lead to advanced levels of clinical skill and practice. For these and a number of other distinctions, it is inappropriate to lump nursing into a general category of health-related occupations or to conclude that nursing's problems are the same as others. There are quantitative and qualitative issues in nursing education that require unique approaches unlike those of any other clinical health providers.

In order to provide sufficient numbers of clinical nurses prepared for the diversity of roles required in our emergent health care system, it is essential that some form of federal support be continued. At the same time, it is entirely appropriate that allocations among programs be reviewed objectively and regularly. Significant economies could be realized if nursing would order its own educational house aright. If all preparatory and advanced programs in nursing were located in collegiate systems, if all the overly small programs were terminated and larger programs

*A later agreement provided for approval of NTA funds at the $103 million level.

expanded to achieve an economy of scale, if articulated programs were instituted so as to reduce loss of time and money in the advancement of career mobility, if statewide and regional planning were utilized to avoid unnecessary duplication of effort, if greater cooperation and sharing of scarce resources, both human and capital, were undertaken then American nursing could present an irrefutable claim for public and private support throughout its educational enterprise. Each unresolved internal issue, however, weakens the claim of the whole system and inevitably reduces the probability of comprehensive support matched to appropriate programs.

As helpful as federal funding has been over the past decade—and before—it has also served to hinder important elements in nursing education. The allocation of funds to hospital schools of nursing, for example, at the very time that professional, educational, and socioeconomic determinants were arguing for their dissolution has simply exacerbated and prolonged a problem that might otherwise have been solved. The generalized support of all institutions for preparatory training meant also that marginal facilities found practical arguments for remaining open and even expanding their student bodies.

Over the coming years, public support of nursing at various governmental levels will continue to be needed. It is, in fact, essential to an adequate health care system for the nation. It is hoped, however, that there will emerge a comprehensive blueprint for American nursing education that will develop goals and priorities truly reflecting the needs of the citizens *and* the profession in a balanced, rational way. With that as a given and with the elimination of the current cross-purposes and internal arguing, there is no reason to fear that the public will fail in its response to reasonable requests for support.

REFERENCES

1 "Educational Preparation for Nurse Practitioners and Assistants to Nurses: A Position Paper," American Nurses' Association, New York, 1965.
2 See, for example, "Appendix F. Summary of Recommendations," *An Abstract for Action: Appendices,* McGraw-Hill Book Company, New York, 1971, pp. 123–128.
3 Dorothy Jean Novello, "In Unity—and Diversity—There Is Strength," Editorial, *NLN News,* September 1976.
4 Thelma Schorr, "More in Common than in Conflict," Editorial, *American Journal of Nursing* **74:**1 (January 1974).
5 Andrew K. Dolan, "The New York State Nurses' Association 1985 Proposal: Who Needs It?" *Journal of Health Politics, Policy and Law* 2(4):510–513 (Winter 1978).
6 Ibid., pp. 508–517.
7 "Reconstitute Nursing Board, Panel to Urge," *Arkansas Gazette,* Little Rock, December 28, 1978, p. 4a.
8 Josephine Goldmark, *Nursing and Nursing Education in the United States,* The Macmillan Company, New York, 1923, pp. 194–195.
9 "Appendix F. Summary of Recommendations," *An Abstract for Action: Appendices.*
10 Jerome P. Lysaught, "From Diploma School to College: Two Case Histories on Changing Patterns Within Institutions for Nursing Education," in Jerome P. Lysaught (ed.),

Action in Nursing: Progress in Professional Purpose, McGraw-Hill Book Company, New York, 1974.

11 Jerome P. Lysaught, *You Can Get There from Here: The Orange County/Long Beach Experiment in Improved Patterns of Nursing Education,* The University of Rochester, Rochester, N.Y., 1979.

12 Jerome P. Lysaught, "The Diploma Nurse, the Hospital School, and the National Commission." In Lysaught (ed.), *Action in Nursing.*

13 Jerome P. Lysaught, *From Abstract into Action,* McGraw-Hill Book Company, New York, 1973, chap. V.

14 Stuart H. Altman, *Present & Future Supply of Registered Nurses,* U.S. Department of Health, Education, and Welfare Publication NIH 72–134, 1971.

15 Lysaught (ed.), *Action in Nursing,* p. 240.

16 "Report of the Task Force to Study the Implications of the Recommendations Presented in *An Abstract for Action,*" in Lysaught (ed.), *Action in Nursing,* pp. 121–122.

17 Novello, op. cit.

18 "Resolution 58: Increasing Accessibility of Career Mobility Programs in Nursing," American Nurses' Association House of Delegates Resolution, Biennial Convention, 1978.

19 Preliminary findings of the Western Interstate Commission on Higher Education study of state nursing resources and requirements provided by Dr. Eugene Levine, chief, Manpower Analysis and Resources Branch, Division of Nursing, U.S. Department of Health, Education, and Welfare, 1978.

20 Helen K. Grace, "The BSN as Mandatory Threshold to Nursing Practice: Implications for Graduate Nursing Education," College of Nursing, University of Illinois, Urbana, October 12, 1978 (Mimeographed).

21 Lysaught, *You Can Get There from Here.*

22 Patricia T. Haase, *A Proposed System for Nursing: Theoretical Framework,* Part 2, Southern Regional Education Board, Atlanta, 1976.

23 Mary W. Searight, "A Tentative Proposal for a New Department of Nursing," Sonoma State College, Sonoma, Calif., December 1971 (Mimeographed).

24 Lysaught, *You Can Get There from Here.*

25 Gloria Ann Hagopian, "The Nursing Deanship: Administrative Problems and Educational Needs," unpublished doctoral dissertation, The University of Rochester, Rochester, N.Y., 1979.

26 *Progress Report on Nurse Training,* Report to the President and the Congress, U.S. Department of Health, Education, and Welfare, 1970.

27 *Nurse Training Act of 1964: Program Review Report,* U.S. Department of Health, Education, and Welfare Public Health Service Publication 1740, 1967.

28 *NTA Digest: Nurse Training Act of 1971,* U.S. Department of Health, Education, and Welfare NIH Publication 73–311, 1973.

29 Gwynn C. Akin and Josh R. Hogness, "Trends in Financing Higher Education, Health Education, and Nursing Education," keynote address at a seminar cosponsored by the American Association of Colleges of Nursing and the National League for Nursing Council of Baccalaureate and Higher Degree Programs, Sun Valley, Idaho, July 24, 1977.

30 Haase, op. cit., pp. 1–11.

31 William K. Selden, "Just One Big Happy Family," *Health Alliance* 1(2):8 (September 1969).

32 Inez G. Hinsvark (director), "The Study of Credentialing in Nursing: A New Approach," *Report of the Committee for the Study of Credentialing in Nursing to the American Nurses' Association,* The University of Wisconsin—Milwaukee, January 1979.

33 Personal communication from Sister M. Fenton Joseph, program coordinator, Division of Nursing, Gwynedd-Mercy College, to Jerome P. Lysaught, dated July 13, 1979.

34 Rose Marie Chioni and E. Schoen, "Preparing Tomorrow's Nurse Practitioner," *Nursing Outlook* 18(10):50 (October 1970).

35 Laura C. Dustan, "A Design for Articulation: A New Approach to Increasing Opportunities for Baccalaureate Nursing Education," University of Iowa College of Nursing, Ames, Iowa, undated (Mimeographed).

36 Haase, op. cit., p. 78–79.

37 Lysaught, *You Can Get There from Here.*

38 Valencia Prock, "Implications for Nursing Education and Practice," paper presented at Conference on Education of Nurses for Public Health, May 23–25, 1973.

39 Haase, op. cit., p. 47.

40 Ibid., p. 45.

41 Lucile A. Wood, *Career Models for Nurse Practitioners,* University of California at Los Angeles, Division of Vocational Education, Report of USDE Grant 8-0627, March 1972.

42 *Progress Report on Nurse Training.*

43 *NTA Digest: Nurse Training Act of 1971.*

44 Judith Jezek, "Financing Nursing Education: Past and Future," graduate research paper, The University of Rochester, Rochester, N.Y., Spring 1979.

45 American Nurses' Association News Release, dated January 22, 1979, issued from the Washington, D.C., office of the ANA.

46 "Veto of NTA Points Profession to Edge of Crisis," *American Journal of Nursing* **79** (4):569ff. (April 1979).

47 Cheryl M. Fields, "Cuts Sought in Student Aid, Health-Education Programs," *Chronicle of Higher Education,* January 29, 1979, p. 4.

Chapter 6

Implementation of the Recommendations for Nursing Careers

One of the most pervasive and perplexing problems examined by the National Commission for the Study of Nursing and Nursing Education (NCSNNE) was that of the nursing shortage throughout the United States a decade ago. At that time, the conventional wisdom argued that increasing the number of nursing students together with expanding the categories of aides, attendants, and assistants would ensure adequate care to meet clients' needs. The National Commission was skeptical. An examination of past efforts as well as then current attempts to solve the problem through these means was less than reassuring. The emphasis on "fresh inputs" and "helping personnel" seemed, if anything, to exacerbate the single most powerful cause of the shortage of nurses—the lack of retention.

Continued study of the supply of nurses since 1968 confirms the fact that about one out of every four registered nurses does not even maintain a license and another 25 percent are inactive [1]. Perhaps one out of every three of the employed nurses actually works on a part-time basis—thus leaving some 35 percent of our total registered nurse population to meet all the needs for practice, education, administration, and the varied responsibilities of a changing health care system. In addition, there are significant rates of turnover among nursing personnel which magnify the problems of staffing—and, of course, geographic, clinical, and functional specialty maldistribution that further complicates the situation.

At the same time, it is important to recognize that the nursing shortage is also a state of mind, a social perception over and above a manpower reality. In 1979, for example, an advisory panel on the nurse shortage was established by the American Hospital Association (AHA). This body received the results of two surveys conducted by the AHA staff within weeks of each other. In the first study, only hospital associations were queried and 18 state groups reported a "critical" shortage of nurses. In the second survey, a few state nurses' associations as well as all the state hospital associations were asked about their manpower situation. This time, 36 out of 45 states reported a considerable shortage of nurses whereas 28 state hospital associations (a gain of 10) reported they were having a "critical" shortage. Closer examination of the information indicated that six states had returned replies from both nurses' and hospital associations; there was agreement in three cases, direct disagreement in the other three [2]. Within any given state, moreover, there may be found sharp differences between rural and metropolitan sections, between affluent and impoverished communities.

One thing, however, that seems safe in this welter of information and misinformation is the statement that were all of the registered nurses resident in this country to return to full-time professional activity, there would be no shortage that could not be met, no need that could not be filled. It is this paradox that causes econometricians, on the one hand, to say there is no nursing shortage while administrators and nursing service directors, on the other hand, bemoan unfilled, budgeted positions and look for contingencies to meet their staffing problems. To bridge these gaps will require far more than cosmetic treatment.

In 1970, the National Commission argued forcefully for an examination of root factors and the planning of career opportunity and reward systems that would retain our best nurses within care settings. The very fact that the nursing shortage occupies so much of our time today is proof that the process is still incomplete; the question at hand is whether we have made progress toward solving the underlying causes of that shortage. One should not ignore the sources of supply, but the factors affecting retention are much more authoritative in determining the adequacy of our response to health care provision. It would take us over 6 years, for example, to graduate the number of registered nurses, at present rates, simply to equal the number of R.N.s who have dropped their licenses. This kind of gap, of course, can never be made up unless we determine why persons abandon nursing careers and how we can develop longer commitments and more active patterns of professional performance.

PLANNING FOR NURSING CAREERS

One of the obvious stumbling blocks to a more lengthy career in nursing lies in the lack of systematic planning for the utilization of nurses and for the encouragement of professional growth and development. In 1968, it seemed that most studies of health personnel saw nursing as an undifferentiated manpower bloc. Projections for numbers of nurses needed were based largely on the number of institutions—hospitals, nursing homes, educational programs, etc.—in a given political division. Invariably, the answers lay in some increased number of "nurses" with almost no defined characteristics of specialty practice, preparatory level, or role expectations. A nurse was a nurse was a nurse—and presumably held the innate capacity of an assembly line fitting to serve as an interchangeable part.

To add to these problems, many planning agencies, such as the National Advisory Commission on Health Manpower, did not include nurses on their decision-making bodies. This exclusion of nurses tended to ensure that only the most traditional, and usually restrictive, views of the nursing profession would be applied to projections for the rearrangement of responsibilities and functions. In short, most planning efforts suffered from a global, undifferentiated approach to the assessment of needs for nurse personnel coupled too often with sharply limited input from the persons who might have represented the emergent characteristics of the profession that could enhance the total delivery of health care in this country.

As a basic solution to this problem, the National Commission recommended that nurses be appointed to all groups involved in health care planning at all levels —federal, state, county, and region—and, in addition, that the federal Division of Nursing continue and expand its studies on differentiated nursing needs so that future health planning groups might have better information on the infrastructure of the profession and its relationship to varied role expectations and client care requirements [3]. Beginning with the Secretary's Committee to Study Extended Roles for Nurses in 1971, the Department of Health, Education, and Welfare (HEW) has fostered a much more active involvement of nursing in planning and advisory committees across the whole range of concerns for health maintenance, disease reduction, and episodic intervention. Nurses have been admitted to membership in the prestigious Institute of Medicine of the National Academy of Sciences and to panels of the National Institutes of Health. Special government programs were designed to encourage and train nurse practitioners with advanced clinical skills and to foster nurse physician interaction in the planning and presentation of such programs. In numbers and in ratios, the nursing input may still be small and highly selective, but precedents have been established and, in the opinion of this study staff, a significant opportunity has been presented.

Just as important, in response to a provision of the Nurse Training Act of 1975, the Division of Nursing launched four independent studies of the requirements for future nursing manpower needs embodying analyses of differentiated levels and expanded roles in clinical settings [4]. These models allow for projections based on the continuation of the present care system, the impact of selective mixes and levels of nursing personnel geared to assessed patient care needs, the probable impact of system dynamics such as expanded health maintenance organizations and their demand for different nurse skills, and the effect that such sweeping changes as enactment of national health insurance might have on manpower requirements.

Through an examination of regional needs and planned changes in approaches to delivering care, health service agencies can selectively extrapolate information from one or more of the models to predict more precisely than in the past not only how many nurses, but with what specialties and levels of clinical expertise, are needed to make the emergent system viable. As we move toward more comprehensive approaches to maintaining health, these new formulations for manpower planning in nursing will become even more significant. At the moment, however, they all support the position that a nursing shortage really does not exist in terms of simplistic number formulas; on the other hand, there is agreement about a lack of nurses prepared to practice at advanced clinical levels which will become more acute with every proposed expansion of the health care delivery system.

The concept of planning throughout the federal system has been fostered by the recommendations of the National Commission and the example of the Department of Health, Education, and Welfare. Some 32 states have established statewide master planning committees since 1970, and planning activities have been assisted by the establishment of joint medical-nursing practice committees in 41 states. These activities, in turn, have encouraged more local and regional planning below the state level. The Health Service Agencies, for example, which have been designated throughout the nation to plan and coordinate health care delivery systems, have for the most part included nurses on their professional panels—though in numbers and proportions far below those of physicians and health administrators.

One of the anecdotal findings of this study staff was the frequent mention—by nurses and nonnurses alike—that nurse membership on planning committees was often limited by the reticence of these representatives to speak up forcefully on issues and by the fact that many lacked advanced clinical skills themselves so that their own position on expanded role expectations was clouded. For the future, then, individuals for appointment to planning agencies and boards should be thoughtfully screened for assertiveness—not belligerence—and clinical expertise. Limited observation of committees that included nurse representatives with these qualities certainly encourages the viewpoint that physicians, administrators, and lay people do listen to nurses who are competent in and capable of articulating the care needs and changing roles of their professional practitioners.

At an even more specific level, it is only fair to suggest that nurses entering into the planning of new departures in care delivery have the advantage of a carefully considered position and rationale for any changes their professional groups might be advocating. In terms of planning for emergent roles in nursing, our staff surveyed all the state nurses' associations to determine whether they had taken formal positions on several issues that relate to clinical practice and to the differentiation of nurse roles. We were more concerned to see whether some definitive action—position paper, policy, standard, or official statement—had been taken and disseminated than in the particulars of that action. The summary of our replies is presented in Table 6-1. Each of the four selected issues has been argued in public forums for years, but it is evident that 80 percent or more of these state associations have chosen to remain silent on matters that their own members and leaders regard as critical.

Another oft-cited anecdotal fact about nursing is that no issue is ever presented before a legislative or administrative panel regarding the future of the profession without having the most vociferous advocates and opponents emerge from the ranks of nursing itself. Whether this is the cause or the consequence of inaction of the professional associations at the state and local levels is a matter to ponder. Its impact on the planning process is predictable—and problematic. Any of the models devel-

Table 6-1   Number of State Nursing Associations Taking Definitive Action Supporting Professional Nursing Issues

Professional nursing issue	Yes	No
Diversified levels of R.N. licensure	2	49
Clinical specialization certification	10	41
Clinical competence for relicensure	3	48
B.S. degree as a basis for professional designation	7	44

oped through the Division of Nursing require basic definitions of differentiated levels and clinical competency. In the absence of an agreed professional definition by nursing, even the best-intentioned agencies and committees are unable to determine effective ways to utilize nurses in a changing care environment.

This may be why state nurses' associations rate health planning as one of their greatest opportunities in terms of professional thrust and also rate the development of a "united nursing" as one of the greatest challenges to the future of the profession. On the future agenda of all nursing organizations must lie the necessity to develop common definitions and policies to provide guidance and parameters to planning bodies seeking to integrate these practitioners into a new system of care, cure, and health delivery.

In the parlance of those who study group dynamics in organizations, the situation in nursing is unfrozen with regard to planning. More nurses are involved in federal, state, and regional health planning and policy groups than ever before. The limitations on an enlargement of this participative base are largely dependent upon the quality of the clinical expertise that nursing can bring to bear on health problems, the ability of the individual members to work vigorously and harmoniously with other representatives toward an improved health care system, and the capacity of nursing, through its various organizations and associations, to achieve a common purpose and direction concerning the future career expressions of the profession. For once, the problems are mostly internal; success or failure turns on nurses and nursing. The credit or the blame is nursing's alone to garner. The probability is weighted toward success, but professional leadership must continue to be exerted if the early promise is to be realized.

RETENTION OF QUALIFIED PRACTITIONERS

In 1970 [5] and 1973 [6] the National Commission for the Study of Nursing and Nursing Education mustered evidence to show that nursing suffered from critical deprivations in terms of motivators that could retain its most qualified and capable people in patient care. Using the theories of Maslow [7] and Herzberg [8], the Commission's staff demonstrated that nursing found it difficult to realize even the security level of needs satisfaction—which essentially is a hygiene factor that merely prevents dissatisfaction while not leading to motivated, goal-directed behavior. Beyond the security level, nurses found that inducements were essentially designed to take them away from client care into either education or administration. To overcome the combined impact of these pressures, the Commission proposed both economic and organizational improvements. Without change and substantial amelioration of these conditions, it is fatuous to speak of career perspectives or the retention of qualified clinical practitioners. In 1978–1979, this study staff attempted to assess the long-term implementation of these recommendations.

Economic Security in Nursing

One of the most controversial developments of the sixties and early seventies was the growth of collective bargaining in nursing. Despite the fact that women tend to be less favorable to unionization than men are [9], the growth of collective bargaining was encouraged by nursing's own professional organizations at the national and state levels and was accelerated by the impetus of outside organizers from traditional unions for professional workers and health employees.

There are a multiplicity of reasons for seeking recognition and bargaining rights, but the National Commission had pointed out that a very basic problem for nursing lay in the inadequate salaries and unsatisfactory working conditions that prevailed in health care institutions, agencies, and offices across the country. When nursing salaries were compared with median full-time earnings for women in a variety of occupations, they fell far behind professional and technical fields requiring comparable education and responsibility. Nurses barely exceeded clerical and office workers in terms of salary and lagged behind teachers, librarians, social and recreation workers, and many other health service personnel.

Indeed, many of the half million "nurses" who no longer maintain a license to practice may be found in the full-time labor force in nonnursing occupations that command a substantially greater salary along with improved working conditions and perquisites. Another half million who retain licenses undoubtedly find the economic situation so unattractive that they are content to remain totally inactive in terms of the practice of their profession. So complete is the depression of salary levels for nursing that it has been described by economists as an inelastic occupation—meaning that normal increments of 4 or 5 percent in salary have no attractive power since the overall base is too low to induce anyone to enter even part-time work for the additional sums that might be involved.

Table 6–2 displays the change in nursing salaries over the past 20 years in terms of reported median earnings of professional nurses at the staff nurse level. Between 1959 and 1969, there was a 73 percent growth rate; between 1969 and 1979, there

Table 6-2 Median Full-Time Earnings for Registered Nurses in Hospital Settings, 1959–1979

Year	Median full-time earnings
1959	$ 3,819
1969	6,632
1979	12,480

was an 88 percent growth rate. Overall, nursing salaries have more than tripled over the 23 year period, but the combined effect of inflation and concurrent increases to comparison groups has done little to affect the relative ranking of registered nurses on an economic scale. This situation can perhaps be best illustrated in the case of hospital nursing. In Figures 6–1 and 6–2, we can see comparisons of L.P.N. and R.N. salaries over the period from 1971 to 1978 as well as the growth rate of comparative increases for the two occupational groups. Although registered nurses increased their average hourly salary over this period by more than 45 percent, they actually lost in terms of any comparative advantage over licensed practical nurses, whose average salary increased more than 61 percent. Whereas L.P.N.s earned

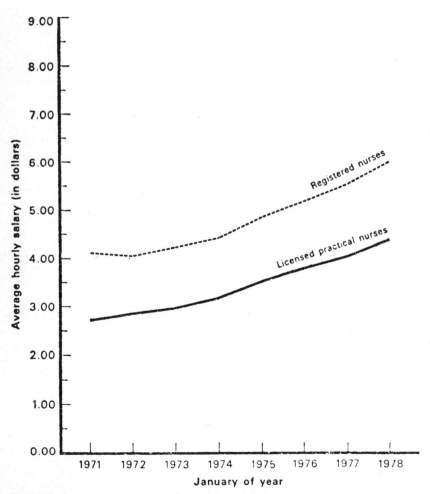

Figure 6–1   Comparison of L.P.N. and R.N. salaries, January 1971–1978. *(From the American Hospital Association. Used with permission.)*

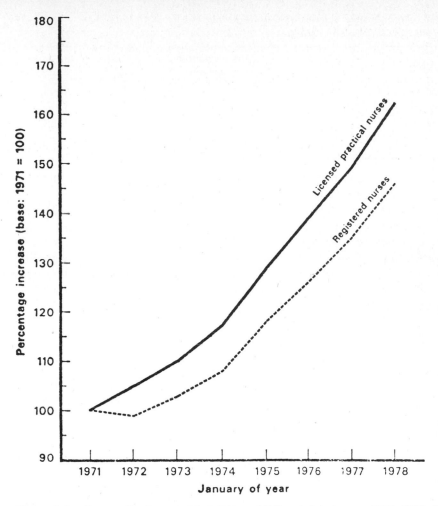

Figure 6–2   Comparative increases in L.P.N. and R.N. salaries, January 1971–1978. *(From the American Hospital Association. Used with permission.)*

almost 66 percent as much as registered nurses at the beginning of this period, they were earning 73 percent as much at the end of the comparison—and the projections would seem to indicate further closure in the coming months and years.

More encouraging in the overall analysis of where we are and where we are headed is the fact that differential salaries within the clinical fields of nursing are beginning to show the impact of expanded role expectancies and increased responsibility. In Table 6–3, we can see a greater distinction than could have been found in 1968 in the reporting of registered nurses' salaries within the clinical setting. A much more detailed examination must be given to the costs of advanced education, training, and certification in order to establish the economic return truly represented by increased salaries for advanced practitioners, but the beginning distinctions are

Table 6-3   Comparative Salaries of Differentiated
Nursing Positions in the Hospital Setting, 1978

Position	Reported mean full-time salary
Nurse anesthetist	$20,364
Nurse specialist	17,724
Head or charge nurse	16,500
Clinical team leader	14,040
Staff nurse	12,480

significant for their confirmation of changes in roles and positions in the changing delivery patterns for patient care.

By any analysis, the salary levels and patterns in nursing represent inadequate figures in comparison with those of other females, other health workers—particularly males—and other occupations of similar preparation and responsibility. To some extent, this condition mirrors the general depression of female compensation in our society. The National Commission on Working Women, for example, argues that women in the same job category as men generally earn 45 to 65 percent of the male salary dollar [10]. This, of course, in turn reflects the fact that job advancement and responsibilities have long been skewed in our society.

The basic question is whether the economics practiced by our health care industry can serve to keep not just enough nurses in practice, but our best and brightest nurses serving in such a capacity. The answer is harsh, but must be faced. At present, nurses can receive more money for taking nonpractitioner positions in education or administration with a substantial improvement in working conditions: reduced shift work, more benefits, increased latitude. Moreover, nurses can enter alternative fields in community, public, and school health and find more pleasant and better-paying positions even though many of these arenas actually tend to restrict the nurse from practicing to full capacity because of various regulations and traditional perceptions.

The gains achieved by nursing over the past 20 years have been impressive in terms of previous earnings, but not in terms of real dollars or purchasing power. There is evidence that health care institutions can reap actual economic benefits from increasing their registered nursing staff, paying higher salaries, encouraging expanded practice, and reducing both withdrawal and turnover. It is essential that health care administrators and other care practitioners, particularly physicians, examine objectively the contribution of nurses to patient care and assess this on the basis of what is a fair return on social performance, rather than developing increments on an inadequate base founded on arbitrary and capricious salary determinations of the past.

Job Satisfaction in Nursing

Over and beyond the matter of basic economic security, there is a great need to examine the intrinsic job satisfactions that are attached to the practice of nursing. The reasons have been well-documented, but bear brief repetition:

1   Despite the fact that an overwhelming number of nurses chose their profession in order to "care for people," it is a fact that they spend more time in non-nursing functions than in patient ministration [11].

2   As nurses assume more responsibility in service institutions, their work becomes even more concentrated on organizational matters and less involved with patient care. Thus, the traditional patterns for nursing careers frustrate the concept of clinical growth around client concerns [12].

3   Finally, the increasing discontinuity between the intrinsic desires of the individual nurse to practice clinical skills and the need of the traditional system to develop administrative behaviors has forced a choice between conformity and withdrawal [13].

As the National Commission observed in 1973, "It has been ironic that in nursing one could find recognizable career paths in administration or education, but not in the practice of client care itself." To overcome this problem, *An Abstract for Action* called for the development of career patterns in clinical practice such that rewards and promotions would be based on excellence in providing care and that increased responsibility would take the form of clinical direction and care leadership rather than systems maintenance.

Since 1973, an increasing number of institutions and agencies have attempted to reorganize nursing service in order to establish a career pattern for practitioners in the spirit of the Commission's recommendations. In our survey of hospitals, for example, over 60 percent of the respondents indicated that recognition, reward, and responsibility are now essentially related to clinical competence within their nursing service. Whereas the traditional hierarchy of the hospital militated against the use of a supervisory nurse for patient care—only 7 percent of a supervisor's time was spent in direct patient care—the respondents to our survey indicate that significant shifts have taken place at this level. Approximately 73 percent of all the institutions replying to our questionnaire now expect and require their supervisory nurses to be more clinically competent than staff nurses—and give primary consideration to excellence in practice for selection and promotion.

A large majority of the hospitals, 71 percent, reported a significant increase in the proportion of time devoted to patient care by nursing service, and in some hospitals there are efforts under way to develop an entire R.N. care staff so that care can be enhanced and a career pattern based on clinical excellence can be wholly developed. This repatterning of nurse utilization is essential because the reconstruction of roles at the staff, head nurse, and supervisory levels is under way but the acquisition and utilization of nurse practitioners and clinical specialists is still not generalized throughout our care system. Only 27 percent of the reporting hospitals had hired nurse practitioners—largely because of traditional job classifications and budgetary restraints. Approximately 36 percent of the hospitals had moved to designate certain clinical nursing positions as ones that required advanced certification, and slightly more than 33 percent of all the institutions were attempting to restructure the entire salary and compensation structure to encourage the concept of graded levels of clinical competence that would lead to a career pattern centered on patient care.

In order to assess how far these ideas have permeated the entire care system, we asked the state nurses' associations how they viewed the adequacy of the reward system today in terms of both economic and professional realities. Their responses are summarized in Table 6–4. Although these responses, of course, are perceptions, not established "facts," they represent a significant view of the world as seen by the professional associations for nurses.

The mean values for all three elements of the current reward system are seen as largely inadequate, with only a few states registering what could be construed as satisfaction with the status quo. Salary, for reasons discussed earlier, is perceived as the least adequate single factor, but increased professional authority and responsibility are close behind. The development of expanded roles rates the highest mark, a result consistent with the information supplied by our hospital respondents—but the rating only nears the midway point between inadequate and adequate.

By any measure, the feelings represented by the replies of the state nurses' associations must be seriously taken and thoughtfully considered. They tell us that the malaise and dissatisfaction so evident in nursing a decade ago have not been removed and that our current reward systems—though moving in the right direction —are not adequate to retain those nurses who could be the greatest contributors to the enhancement of our health care system. The very human needs for esteem, recognition, and self-actualization are not going to be satisfied where role expansion and professional responsibility are sharply limited or denied.

That there is growing awareness of these issues outside of nursing is evident in the recent report of the American Hospital Association's Advisory Panel on Nurse Shortage. This group agreed that "institutions need to assess the extent to which they satisfy professional nurses' expectations and provide a work environment conducive to professional practice" [14]. In particular, the panel urged each institution to review the quality of commitment held by administration, medicine, and supporting staff to the practice of nursing and the enhancement of professional practice and urged that nurses be involved in the determination of utilization patterns, role expansion, and specialization.

The report of this advisory panel is significant for its emphasis on the need to develop satisfying career patterns and enlightened approaches to clinical utilization and patterning. It is perhaps even more significant in terms of its refusal to accept traditional short-term approaches in the consideration of nursing shortages. There

Table 6–4   Ratings of Elements of the Current Reward System for Nursing by State Nurses' Associations, 1978

Reward	Very adequate 3	Adequate 2	Inadequate 1	Mean $\overline{X}$
Significant salary increments	1	14	36	1.31
Expanded roles and professional challenge	3	18	30	1.47
Increased professional authority and responsibility	2	14	35	1.35

is much that professional nursing would hold in common with the AHA panel; the question, of course, is whether the report will have any impact beyond a certain historic value.

If we are to turn the corner on the road to career satisfaction and practitioner retention in nursing, it will require the support and commitment of health administrators and physicians as well as the best efforts of the nursing profession. For the public, however, to receive the best care from the most capable, it is essential that we retain nurses in practice, compensate them properly for doing so, and remove the traditional limitations we have placed on the role expansion of nursing care. A start has been made; discernible progress can be documented over the past decade. But in 1980 we still have far to go.

RECRUITMENT OF NURSING STUDENTS

Over the period of the National Commission's existence, from 1967 through 1973, there was a dramatic increase in the number of students admitted to R.N. programs. This was due largely to the rapid expansion of associate degree programs, which more than offset the reduction in student numbers caused by the closing of hospital schools. Nevertheless, a more in-depth analysis showed that there was a decline over this same period in the proportion of high school graduates choosing nursing as a career. The "baby boom" following the Second World War accounted for this seeming anomaly because the upsurge in high school graduations meant there were more persons going into nurse training even though the proportion was reduced.

In analyzing these trends, the Commission staff concluded that the increasing range of occupational choice available to female high school graduates—more than a form of rejection of traditional occupations—would impact on both nursing and teaching. There would be both positive and negative consequences. Some students in the past may have gone into nursing simply because it was available. With increased choice, there was greater assurance that selections were truly based on alternative weightings. At the same time, many excellent students who might have opted for a career in nursing now found themselves attracted toward medicine, law, engineering, and a host of other fields that had once been nearly closed to female applicants.

It seemed to the Commission that future recruiting efforts in nursing should stress the growing scientific base of the profession, the opportunities for expanded clinical roles, and the career perspectives for a lengthy and satisfying commitment to practice. This approach would emphasize the intellectual and behavioral components of nursing and would challenge potential students to assume roles of responsibility and authority. To some extent, this approach would be an about-face from the most saccharine recruitment endeavors, which played up the affective elements in the nursing role to the exclusion of the knowledge and skill necessary to execute patient care properly.

As we enter the new era of declining postsecondary populations and college enrollment, the matter of nurse recruitment takes on a larger significance than ever before. As indicated in Figure 6–3, there has been a slight reduction in the number of female high school graduates, and the rapid growth in R.N. admissions has, since 1973, been replaced by an essentially steady state with only small changes from year to year. Internal adjustments continue to be made, with hospital schools closing and associate degree and baccalaureate programs growing only slowly, but total admissions have shown growing stability, with only slight increases, since 1972.

Over the next decade, there will be greater reductions in the number of high school graduates, and the loss to nursing will be compounded if those projections are correct which forecast a declining percentage of these graduates going into

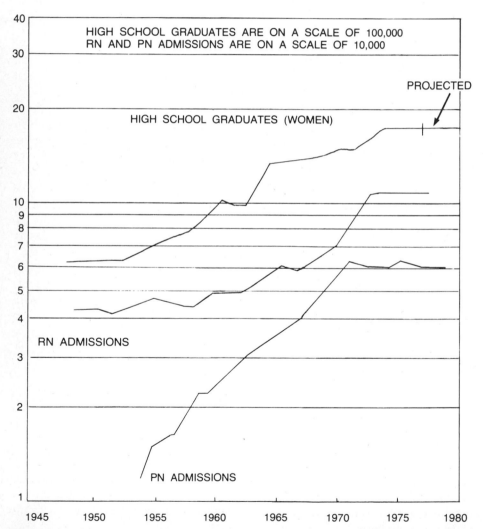

Figure 6–3   Comparison of trends in number of female high school graduates and admission to R.N. and P.N. schools of nursing, 1948–1978. *(From the National League for Nursing. Used with permission.)*

postsecondary educational programs. The impact of affirmative action and antidiscrimination programs will continue to expand the choices for all females so that nursing will have to become more competitive than it has ever been in order to attract the kinds and quality levels it needs in students.

One obvious area in which nursing should expand its efforts is the recruitment of male high school graduates. Traditionally, only 6 or 7 percent of American nursing students are male—many of these being ex-military personnel who served in health care departments. The image of nursing as a female occupation is so pervasive that male high school students seldom consider it as a career choice. It must be added, however, that no counterpart group has ever actively sought to encourage applications from and acceptance of males into nursing as has been done in encouraging females into medicine. The National Student Nurses' Association and other groups have developed recruitment materials and pamphlets aimed at potential male applicants, but the general response has been quite low.

Actually, the issue is more far-reaching than it appears. The sexual stereotyping of any profession is an anachronism. In the health care fields it is a disservice to the client population which the professions have no right to impose. The belated efforts of medicine to increase the number of women admitted to its schools have brought into their training programs a whole new pool of intelligent and caring people. By the same token, when nursing is even more skewed on this same dimension, it is failing to exercise its professional responsibility to seek out the best applicants— whomever and wherever they may be.

When medicine, law, and engineering were virtually closed to females, there may have been some justification for the reluctance with which many nurse educators and service directors viewed the admittance of men to the profession. But affirmative action should cut both ways. If male students could see the vision of a full, unambiguous profession for patient care, complete with a scientific base to guide its practice, with expanded roles and joint collaboration with medicine, then a whole new dimension might be added to their conception of nursing. If it is perceived as a true discipline with rigorous requirements and a strong commitment to enhanced care and evaluated outcomes, then there would be a good likelihood of its attracting increased numbers of males. Once a "critical mass" were established, further expansion would develop along natural lines.

Aside from its signal failure in the immediate past to attract male students, however, nursing must be commended for its earnest and largely successful attempts to increase the numbers of minority students admitted into preparatory programs. The National Student Nurses' Association mounted a national campaign in the seventies to attract all kinds of minority students into the profession. The National League for Nursing (NLN) and the American Nurses' Association (ANA) actively supported these efforts, as well as undertaking actions of their own to bring minority peoples into the profession. Individual schools and colleges also provided assistance and tailored forms of programming to ensure that applicants were given every opportunity for admission and successful completion of their preparatory training. Nursing would agree that still more effort is required in these directions, but its record of achievement is unmistakable. Discrimination as a pejorative is almost nonexistent in American nursing—its last true vestige being the lack of males within the ranks.

One problem that continues to surface in site visits and interviews, however, deserves particular mention. It was noted in 1968 and still is mentioned today. This is the matter of counseling and information given to high school students particularly, but sometimes also to individuals considering a second career. Many high school and vocational counselors seem to be unaware that there are four preparatory tracks into nursing, including three routes to the R.N. license. Little substantive information is provided to students seeking guidance on where to apply; differences between and among programs are not explained; and such concerns as accreditation, attrition, and achievement on licensure examinations are frequently dismissed.

Counselors, of course, cannot reasonably be expected to know each occupational field thoroughly. The Department of Labor some time ago identified more than 120 different health occupations alone, and these were designated by some 250 occupational titles. But it should be a matter of continuing concern to the National League for Nursing and the American Nurses' Associations, as well as their state groups and constituent bodies, to provide up-to-date materials that can assist both the counselor and the potential student in assessing the alternative paths into nursing. In a recent study of nursing students, Bullough and Sparks found that the reason given more frequently than any other for choosing a particular school was its proximity; the curriculum or philosophy of the school ranked well down the list [15]. This method of choice suggests that a broad generalization about the sameness of preparatory nursing programs is still operative, and, for the sake of the student and the profession, this perception should be altered. An informed choice at the outset would help reduce attrition and certainly assist satisfactory career goal achievements for the nursing student.

NEW SOURCES OF MANPOWER SUPPLY

In 1970, the National Commission urged nursing to expand its recruitment efforts not only toward men and societal minorities, but also toward selected groups of "advantaged" people: graduates of baccalaureate programs in the arts and sciences who were looking for a vocational career, graduates of advanced degree programs in the biological and social sciences who might find more satisfaction in an applied science that could use their knowledge base in furthering patient care, and mature men and women who were essentially seeking a second career after, perhaps, rearing a family and having pursued another line of employment successfully.

As a result of the economic recession of the past several years and its effect, in turn, on employment opportunities, schools of nursing have found more and more applicants from the first two categories whereas associate degree programs, in particular, seem to be sought out by individuals in the third category. As one means of comparing the activity of the institutions in this area, approximately 49 percent of all of our responding schools had established planned programs to attract and admit minority students, whereas only 18 percent of the institutions had similar programs for students from the arts and sciences. On closer examination, however, this latter figure may not be truly representative. Over 20 percent of the baccalaureate programs *did* have programs to aid in the admittance of students and graduates from other disciplines, whereas only 14 percent of the associate degree programs had mounted such an effort. Since, by definition, these individuals would have completed most or all of their college programs, it is only natural that their chief attraction might be to a baccalaureate or higher degree program in nursing. Because of proximity, finances, and the attractiveness of the program, however, a considerable number of these students are willing to begin their nursing careers through an associate degree institution.

A number of the schools of nursing appended statements to their survey forms saying that it was not necessary to establish a special program for arts and science students: the schools simply encouraged applications and provided individualized help in placement and program planning. In other words, they have had sufficient experience over the past few years so that arts and science graduates are not unusual applicants and can be handled through normal processing.

In 1970, the National Commission did comment on the fact that only one school of nursing offered a master's degree in nursing as a first professional degree for prior graduates of baccalaureate programs in other disciplines. The few other schools of nursing at that time with extensive experience in admitting these students simply offered a second baccalaureate degree. Little has changed in this pattern, although Case-Western Reserve University is experimenting with a doctoral program for graduates of other disciplines who will be earning their first degree in nursing at this advanced level and other innovative programs are currently under consideration. It seems to this study staff that the New York Medical College program that pioneered the use of the master's degree as the first professional credential amply demonstrated both the quality and the attractiveness of such an approach. More widespread use of the preparatory master's degree in nursing would provide an added inducement to qualified arts and science majors to enter nursing; the program could be quite rigorous, but it would not suffer the image problems of a return to undergraduate study.

Development from Within

Although nursing has done much to encourage and accept both disadvantaged and advantaged minorities, unquestionably the greatest source of a "new manpower supply" resides within the profession itself. Approximately three out of every four graduates of our current preparatory nursing programs come from a nonbaccalaureate level. Current manpower projections indicate that we may already have reached optimum levels for diploma and associate degree nurses while lagging badly behind the need for baccalaureate and higher degree prepared people [16]. Grace has analyzed a number of alternative proposals for nurse manpower requirements based on various care models developed for the Division of Nursing and has concluded that, if one looks at traditional models and class sizes for nursing education, it would be necessary to develop as many as 850 to 1000 new baccalaureate programs to achieve the numbers and ratios required [17]. This, of course, is a patent impossibility.

What is a real possibility is to confirm what has been done for decades in nursing education, systematize it, and construct an efficient conduit for accomplishing it— the *it* of course being upward mobility from one preparatory level to another. The economies of such an approach practiced on a broad basis would be incredible. It takes only half as long to move an associate degree nurse through a baccalaureate program as it does to admit a novice at the freshman level. Much of the heavy expense of clinical preceptorship has already been invested in the associate degree student so that faculty-student ratios can be reexamined in the light of the student's license to practice. Most important of all, to both the profession and the consumer population, is the provision of added career incentives that can reduce withdrawal, enhance retention, and provide thousands of advanced practitioners for patient care.

As illustrated in Figure 6–4, our current system, or nonsystem, for nursing education admits thousands of students every year, the majority of whom find within 1 or 2 years that they have come to a career bottleneck. As discussed earlier in Chapter 5, baccalaureate programs have for years admitted diploma and associate degree graduates, so that, at any given time, half of the "graduate" students in nursing are actually post-R.N. baccalaureate students. From the standpoint of career development and manpower supply, however, the upward movement of individuals from within the system is the only feasible way to provide the number of advanced clinical practitioners needed. From the standpoint of the nursing profession also, the development of a fluid system for upward mobility is perhaps the only guarantee of ever establishing the baccalaureate degree as the professional base for entry into practice.

Our survey of collegiate programs for nursing preparation indicates that in 1978 more than one-third (36 percent) of the baccalaureate institutions provided special entry programs for associate degree graduates. Moreover, over three-quarters (76 percent) of the associate degree programs reported either planned programs to admit L.P.N.s or integrated programs in which the L.P.N. program essentially mirrored the first year of the A.D.N. program. Thus, there are precedents, models, and examples already in place. With proper statewide planning, it would be possible within less than 5 years to have organized, articulated preparatory programs across the country so that nurses who wish to and have the capacity and initiative could move up to increasing levels of clinical competence and responsibility.

There are any number of positive reasons, both societal and professional, for advancing practitioners up within the system, but it may well be that economic determinism will settle the issue in favor of articulation. With a reduced college-age population and with the competition from an increasing number of professions and occupations seeking female applicants, the baccalaureate institutions for nursing education may well recognize that the more than 800,000 nurses with diploma or associate degree preparation are simply too attractive a financial resource to ignore. With the contemporary growth of mandatory continuing education, too, the nonbaccalaureate students may find it much more advantageous to pursue an integrated sequence leading to a degree rather than simply accumulate continuing education units or credits. Thus, a confluence of many pressures argues for the systematic development of recruitment from within nursing for the next several years.

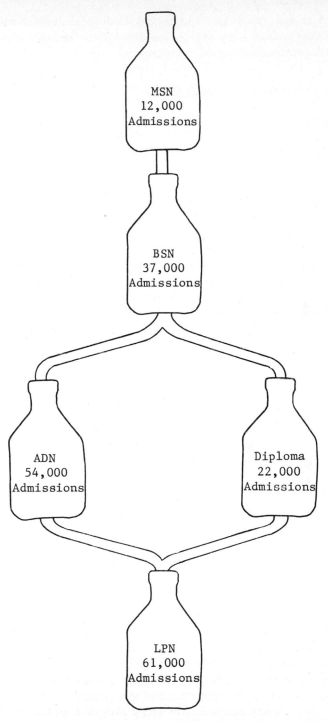

Figure 6–4 Schematic diagram of admissions to various nursing levels in 1978.

Among other things, this reorganization could end for all time the debate about a nursing shortage by ensuring that sufficient numbers of the right kinds, levels, and specialties are provided across the country.

LICENSURE AND CAREER PERFORMANCE

In 1970, the National Commission for the Study of Nursing and Nursing Education examined the growing ferment in the field of licensure and credentialing. At that time, this was an issue throughout the health professions. In some areas, as in medical technology, there was open hostility over the control of registration, with a power struggle developing between the American Society of Medical Technologists and the American Society of Clinical Pathologists. An increasing number of prestigious colleges and universities were objecting to the multiplicity of accrediting agencies, licensing groups, and other bodies that sought to inquire into programs and graduates and to levy fees for these "services." People within the health professions sought to develop equivalency across programs so that horizontal and vertical mobility might be enhanced. The rising voice of consumerism targeted in on the lack of public scrutiny that often accompanied licensure and credentialing.

Although there were problems in nurse licensure, they were generally of a different nature and intensity than those in credentialing of other health occupations, so it seemed to the National Commission that there was no utility to be found in raising issues to a higher level of abstraction than necessary. As a result, we confined ourselves solely to the licensure of nurses and, in doing so, we applied as a first standard of assessment this definition of licensure:

> Licensure is a process by which an agency of government grants formal permission to an individual to practice a given occupation upon determining that the applicant has attained the minimal degree of competency necessary to ensure that the public health, safety, and welfare will be reasonably protected.

The function of the government agency, then, is to represent the public in determining what is minimal competency, how to test or otherwise determine that it has been attained, and how to provide continuing assurance so that health, safety, and welfare are not at hazard.

Over the years, abuses have crept into licensure. In some cases, the government agency actually was composed wholly of the people who were licensed in the occupation they were supposed to regulate. There was an honest question as to whether conflict of interest obtained and whether doubtful cases or procedures would be decided in favor of the public or the occupation. In other cases, it seemed that licensure was used to restrict the number of practitioners of a given occupation and thus by law create an oligopoly. Moreover, licensure procedures can become so embedded in tradition and formalism that they become obsolete unless there are periodic efforts to ensure their currency and significance.

Most of these transgressions on the intent and spirit of licensure were absent in nursing. Of the 51 jurisdictions, most states and the District of Columbia had state licensure boards for nursing that were free-standing agencies established to carry out mandates of the state nurse practice act. In three states these functions were carried out by agencies in the state department of higher education. In most states there were nonnurse members to represent the public's concern, and in all cases there were procedures for review or appeal. In all site visits and interviews conducted by the Commission staff, there was no indication that boards of nursing failed to consider the public or gave unfair priorities to the profession's viewpoints on issues that arose.

In terms of serving to exclude practitioners, there was general agreement that state licensure examinations developed from the test pools of the National League for Nursing were reasonable though, perhaps, a little too traditional in their composition. They were based essentially on the five fields of the medical-hospital model (medicine, surgery, obstetrics, pediatrics, and psychiatric nursing), and some nurse educators, particularly baccalaureate faculty, felt that more content in the examinations should be devoted to emergent practice, such as primary nursing. On discussing this concern with representatives of state boards of nursing, however, our staff was assured that formal proposals for change would be considered and that no specific recommendations had been received to change the basic structure of the test instrument. Indeed, we were told by representatives of several boards that favorable consideration would be given to experimental programs in nursing education and that new tests could be devised or examinations waived for a period of time to allow for the demonstration of competency on the part of graduates. (It should be emphasized that not all boards of nursing would have this freedom of action because of the statutory regulations under which they operated.)

Rates of failure on the state board examinations varied, but nationwide almost one out of five applicants failed to pass the test on first sitting. This substantial number, however, was reduced through retesting following a period of on-the-job experience. In one state selected at random, for example, almost 95 percent of those who failed the first examination received passing scores on reexamination provided that they had actually been employed in a health care setting throughout the intervening period. This finding suggests that many graduates require some form of internship after graduation before they can effectively qualify to pass the state licensure examination. Naturally, some individuals argued that the examinations were too difficult, but the majority felt that preparatory programs should be improved and thereby eliminate high failure rates.

In only one area, however, could we discern a high level of acrimony about failures on the state licensing examinations; this involved the testing of foreign nurse graduates. Many hospitals and some state hospital associations had become involved in recruiting foreign nurse graduates to come to the United States to practice in areas where administrators claimed there was an acute nursing shortage. The failure rate for these individuals was extremely high, and vigorous complaints were lodged on their behalf by administrators and some directors of nursing service who felt that the written examinations placed these foreign graduates at an unfair disadvantage —although any evidence that our staff could gather was sheerly anecdotal in this regard. To deal with this problem and to prevent insofar as possible its spread, a Commission on Graduates of Foreign Nursing Schools was founded and funded by the American Nurses' Association and the National League for Nursing in 1976. With additional money from the Department of Health, Education, and Welfare (HEW) and the W. K. Kellogg Foundation, the Commission has developed tests in both nursing practice and English proficiency and has provided these examinations in some 30 foreign countries in a series of administrations.

Candidates who pass these examinations will receive a certificate to be used as an aid in obtaining visa preference, as an aid in obtaining a work permit, and as a requirement for admission to state boards. It is anticipated that the screening examination not only will reduce the 80 percent failure rate of foreign nurse graduates through its selective processing of applicants, but also will materially reduce the frustrations and disappointments that have occurred in the past when these nurses were admitted nonsystematically into health care institutions and only later discovered that their proficiency in English and/or nursing practice simply could not measure up to prevailing state standards.

In another recent development, the Council of State Boards of Nursing, which had long functioned as an organization in collaboration with the American Nurses' Association, separated entirely from that professional organization and established itself as an independent body. Undoubtedly this was done in part to avoid any appearance of a monopolistic control of licensure. The council will continue to consult and cooperate on matters relating to nurse practice acts, the development of standards for preservice nursing education programs, and providing the policies and the means for licensure examination.

In 1970, the National Commission proposed four specific recommendations relating to nursing licensure: that mandatory licensure replace voluntary licensure in all states, that relicensure include a periodic review of continued competency in practice, that nurse and physician practice acts be couched in flexible terms, and that a single license be retained for the registered nurse and higher levels of practice be recognized through certification. The rationale that linked all these points is simply that the proper role of a government agency is to assure the public of minimum competencies and, beyond this, permit the greatest flexibility and least intrusive controls over the expansion of professional practice and health care delivery.

Voluntary licensure was permitted in some states at the time *An Abstract for Action* was disseminated. This approach to licensure permitted an individual to perform the functions of a registered nurse and to use the title of *nurse* so long as there was no attempt to represent him- or herself as a licensed practitioner. Nurses who wished could take a licensure examination voluntarily and, if successful, could identify themselves as *licensed* or *registered* practitioners. All nurse practice acts now define and protect the use of the title *nurse* and have mandatory licensure requirements for the *registered nurse.* *

The National Commission felt strongly that some form of review for continued clinical competency should be incorporated into relicensure, but there was a strong

---

*Three jurisdictions (Texas, Indiana, and the District of Columbia) have no statutory definition of the scope of nursing practice, whereas Georgia and Oklahoma have provisions that allow exceptions to their licensure regulations. Thus, there are still some shortcomings in the current applications of mandatory licensure.

feeling that the state boards of nursing or the Council of State Boards should properly determine the nature and extent of those procedures. Since 1970, a number of states have mandated continuing education requirements for relicensure in the expectation that such learning will improve clinical competency. Many observers question this assumption, but few have specific suggestions for how to assess continued clinical competence. The American Hospital Association (AHA) Advisory Panel on Nurse Shortage did propose that requirements for relicensure should include demonstrated clinical competency "or, at least, recent employment in a clinical setting" [18]. Conceivably, it would be possible to develop a simple form of institutional documentation to attest to recent clinical experience—though this, of course, is still far from a guarantee of competence. Continuing education, if the requirements are structured so as to stipulate clinical learnings, may be successful. Institutional endorsement might be effective, but it is essential that state boards of nursing address the matter of continuing minimal competency and, perhaps through the council, develop national guidelines for determination and validation of that minimal level.

In approaching the matter of increased flexibility of nurse practice acts and related changes in medical practice acts, the National Commission depended in great part on the success of the National Joint Practice Commission (NJPC) and its state counterpart committees. This reliance was not misplaced. Since 1970, 39 states have enacted or amended their nurse practice acts to permit an expanded nurse role. In some cases, this change in the laws involved the complete rewriting of the practice act itself; in other cases it simply meant the rewriting of board regulations. In still other cases the medical practice act was altered to provide for more delegation by physicians to nurses. Finally, some agency protocols were modified to permit the extension of the nursing role. This overall approach to the legal recognition of new role expectations has likewise been endorsed pragmatically in such documents as the revised standards for nursing services promulgated by the Joint Commission on Accreditation of Hospitals [19]. Although this is a very dynamic field, subject at any time to judicial or agency interpretation, the general analysis is that tremendous progress has been made in the revision of medical and nurse practice acts to accomplish the goals proposed by the National Commission [20].

In terms of the fourth proposal, that of maintaining a single license for registered nurses, licensing procedures have not been altered away from that position although one state has indicated its intention to do so but delayed implementing such a decision. Since 1965, the American Nurses' Association has sometimes used the terms *technical* and *professional* to discriminate between nonbaccalaureate and baccalaureate and higher degree graduates. More recently, in terms of the 1985 resolution, the House of Delegates of the ANA has approved the concept of two levels of registered nursing practice, a *professional* nurse and a nurse *associate*. These groups would be separately defined and licensed, and the baccalaureate level would be required for entry into professional nursing practice.

The National Commission argued forcefully in 1970 that no clear differentiation of competencies could be demonstrated at that time among the graduates of diploma, associate degree, and baccalaureate programs *at the point of entry into practice.* It was therefore not reasonable to have separate licensing procedures, particularly since the primary purpose of licensure is to ensure minimal competency for the protection of the public. Furthermore, the Commission believed that advanced levels of clinical competency should be professionally determined and sanctioned rather than regulated through a government agency.

It is significant to note that the House of Delegates of the ANA passed a companion resolution to establish a mechanism for deriving distinguishing competencies for the proposed two levels of registered nursing. The Commission staff, of course, feels that a more sensible sequence of events would have been, first, to determine whether there truly are differences among graduates at entry level and, then, to pass on whether those differences are sufficient to apply such terms as *professional nurse* to graduates of one preparatory program and withhold it from graduates of other preparatory programs. If differences emerge, as our Commission believed, over time and through experience and continued learning, then clinical classifications should be applied to demonstrated capacity to perform at advanced levels of knowledge and skill.

To this staff, there is no quarrel with the desire, even the necessity, of increasing the professionalism of nursing. We do not, however, believe that licensure should be used as a weapon in the effort to increase the length of preparatory time and the duration of professional socialization. Additionally, we have serious reservations about the resort to government agencies for credentialing of nurses above the minimal level for entry into practice. Already several states have adopted measures to license nurse practitioners or clinical specialists, and there are honest concerns for the impact this trend may have on mobility, endorsement, and relicensure.

On balance, we still recommend the continuance of a single license for registered nursing aimed to ensure the safe practice of entry-level skills. We encourage the professional organizations and specialty practice groups as well as the joint practice committees to pursue actively the development of advanced competency standards and means for determining their accomplishment. We recommend most strongly that nursing itself take responsibility for designating advanced practitioners and for ensuring their continuing competency.

At the same time, when the American Nurses' Association assembles its distinguishing competencies, subject to behavioral demonstration and proven differences, then the Council of State Boards and the various state boards of nursing should examine the evidence objectively and well. If there are significant differences in the entry-level behaviors of preparatory nurse graduates, this should be confirmed properly and legally. Whether the term *professional* should be the operative designation for one group and not for the other is a question about which there should be considerably more reflection and discussion. If one were to apply those terms today, without deviation or grandfathering, perhaps 86 percent of all our nurses would be labeled *not professional.* This staff suspects that different terminology would hasten acceptance of the concept of distinguished entry levels if, indeed, these can be validated and proven.

Meanwhile, the American Nurses' Association has just recently distributed the report of its Study Group on Credentialing in Nursing, which has attempted to formulate definitions, issues, and concerns covering licensure and certification, as well as accreditation and academic recognition through degrees and diplomas [21]. This report and its central recommendation for the creation of a free-standing Nursing Credentialing Center deserves thorough study and consideration before any major changes are proposed in terms of licensure or certification. When things are done in these areas it is best that they be well done, for they can sometimes not be undone—except at great cost and emotional expense.

PROFESSIONAL ORGANIZATION AND NURSING LEADERSHIP

When one considers the potential power and influence of American nursing, it is truly awesome. If one ponders the impact that 2 million people could have on policy development and decision making—even the impact of the 1.5 million who maintain a license—the possibilities are enormous. Having said that, it is necessary to examine the realities of the situation. The American Nurses' Association, the largest of the organizations for American nursing, has a membership of somewhat less than 200,000. This represents about 20 percent of the nurses currently employed in the practice of the profession. Our survey of state nurses' associations indicated slight upward growth since 1970, with the greatest fluctuation occurring in New York, an increase of 12,000, and in California, a decline of 11,000.

The National League for Nursing is essentially composed of institutions and agencies. Individual memberships are on the increase, but it is fair to say that only a few thousand nurses, perhaps 15,000, belong to the NLN although its organizational impact on accreditation, educational programming, and many other areas, including care facilities and agencies, is very great.

It was these two groups, however, that the National Commission had most in mind when it proposed that nursing organizations review their roles and functions to eliminate duplication, develop ways to meet unserved needs, and transfer activities to the most appropriate agency. To an outside observer, it appears that the relationship between and among the organizations for nursing is, if anything, more competitive than it was in 1970. Examples might include:

1   The development of an organization for directors of nursing service within the National League for Nursing which necessarily overlaps the concerns and functions of the ANA Commission on Nursing Services and a third organization of nursing service directors affiliated with the American Hospital Association.

2   The establishment of mechanisms for accrediting and approving continuing education activities by the ANA whereas all other programs in nursing education are accredited through the NLN.

3   The unilateral establishment by the ANA of the Study of Credentialing in Nursing although many of the areas examined have traditionally been under the purview of the NLN.

4   The expansion in influence of the Association of American Colleges of Nursing, which is currently reviewing its structure to consider whether faculty as

well as deans should be members. If the choice is made for inclusion, the impact on the NLN Council of Baccalaureate and Higher Degree Programs would be enormous.

If, however, the National Commission primarily thought of the ANA and NLN in 1970, it was already apparent that a dynamic new element had been introduced into the patterning of nursing organizations. There had been other groups of nurses with common interests for a long while, organizations, for example, of school nurses or public health nurses, but there appeared in the late sixties and early seventies several new groups of specialty practitioners whose primary concern was the strengthening of nurse roles and responsibilities. As indicated in Table 6–5, the growth rate for a number of these groups has been spectacular and, by 1976, their combined numbers were more than half the total membership of the American Nurses' Association—though it should be quickly added that many of the specialty practice group members also belong to the ANA.

More than half of these specialty practice organizations have developed procedures and mechanisms for the certification of advanced clinical practitioners. Relatedly, they provide continuing education opportunities centered on clinical concerns and have encouraged research into nursing practice related to their functional field. Larger organizations offer not only national meetings and programs, but regional services as well. Most of the groups work in collaboration with medical specialties with congruent interests, and, in some cases, joint clinical teaching pro-

Table 6-5   Membership of Specialty Nursing Organizations, 1970–1976

	1970	1973	1976
Association of Rehabilitation Nurses	—	—	945
American Urological Association-Allied	—	228	708
Association of Operating Room Nurses	11,965	16,723	25,045
American Public Health Association	2,970	3,313	1,976
American Association of Nurse Anesthetists	14,539	15,962	17,365
American Association of Nephrology Nurses and Technicians	500	1,500	200
American Association of Neurosurgical Nurses	300	450	750
American Association of Occupational Health Nurses	5,478	6,676	9,000
Emergency Department Nurses' Association	—	5,000	10,000
American Association of Critical Care Nurses	500	12,000	32,000
Orthopedic Nurses' Association	—	1,200	2,835
International Association of Enterostomal Therapists	52	227	710
National Association of Pediatric Nurse Associates and Practitioners	—	200	913
Department of School Nurses/National Educational Association	1,204	1,765	1,850
Nurses' Association of American College of Obstetricians and Gynecologists	3,008	9,962	14,784
Total membership	40,516	75,206	119,081

grams are arranged. Several of the specialty practice groups publish journals that present research findings, new treatment modalities, and articles on professional concerns related to certification and advanced levels of practice.

Since many of these activities, including the development of certification procedures, paralleled the interests of the ANA Divisions on Nursing Practice, the National Commission, in 1973, strongly supported the call by the American Association of Critical-Care Nurses for a meeting of the presidents and executive directors of all organizations essentially composed of nurse members. From that beginning, a Federation of Specialty Nursing Organizations and the ANA was developed and currently consists of some 21 organizations along with a number of auditor groups. The federation meets periodically to discuss common concerns and issues and to exchange information on activities, procedures, and programs.

In 1977, we surveyed the specialty groups that belonged to the federation on their perception of how the cooperative activity was developing. All felt that the current level of organization was essentially preliminary to more definitive progress on mutual goals. Six organizations felt that the group had already made significant strides toward presenting an effective voice of nursing on issues, whereas nine organizations felt that this had not yet been accomplished. All expressed a belief that meetings should be continued and that further progress could be made, but one organization felt strongly that more candor and "real dialogue" were needed to effect mutual confidence and cooperation. Several of the organizations recommended that the federation concept be carried over to the state level through counterpart-type organizations, and our survey of state nurses' association indicates that, in 1978, sixteen states had established such a liaison group while others had established less formal communication lines with the specialty practice groups within the state.

All has not been sweetness and light, however, in the relationships between the ANA and the nurse specialty practice organizations. Particularly in the area of certification there has been disagreement and frustration. At least two specialty practice groups have worked with the ANA Divisions on Practice to develop a joint certification procedure and examination and have subsequently withdrawn to work on the activity by themselves. As a result, there may well be competition between two or more groups seeking to designate and classify advanced levels of practice and to certify the practitioners.

In political terms, too, the federation is more truly described as a confederation. There is no central staff or organization, and between the periodic meetings there may or may not be follow-up on plans or decisions of the members. More important, however, there is no mechanism for setting long-range goals, for assigning priorities, and for planning activities designed to accomplish the ends agreed to by the members. In 1975, the former staff of the National Commission was able to offer the federation a proposal to establish an ad hoc committee on planning, purposes, and structure for the organization along with funding from an outside agency interested in the further professionalization of nursing. To the surprise of the grantor, the proposal was rejected on the basis that this, somehow, might lead to a superorganization of nursing that would be more powerful than any of the participating groups including the American Nurses' Association! At the next meeting of the federation a request to place a reconsideration of the decision on the agenda was rejected, and the question was never again discussed.

It is hard, of course, to understand the reasoning behind the rejection of a committee to examine objectives, plans, and suggestions for structuring a federation of nursing organizations, but the result is an indication that the dream of a House of Nursing is still the victim of parochial concerns, suspicions, and inertia.

At this point, this study staff can only repeat two general recommendations that the National Commission proposed a decade ago:

> **1** That all nursing organizations press forward in their effort to increase cooperation, reduce overlap and conflict, and assign functions to the most capable agency or institution rather than continue parochial behaviors based on self-interest and the protection of "territory."
>
> **2** That individual nurses make a personal and professional commitment by joining and supporting one or more of the organizations which seek to represent them and to speak authoritatively on nursing's contribution to improved health care.

Some time in the future, the American Nurses' Association, the National League for Nursing, the specialty practice organizations, and the many other groups that derive their membership and resources ultimately from individual nurses at the grass roots of this nation must find ways not merely of accommodation, but of cooperation and joint commitment. Until then, the question of who truly speaks for nursing will be unanswerable.

It is inconceivable that nursing, with so many people of intelligence and goodwill, would postpone for much longer the essential need to develop a unified structure that could allow for differences, even value them, but would emphasize the factors that unite rather than divide. Until there is essential unity of purpose, however, nursing will continue as the largest ambiguous profession in American society.

REFERENCES

1 Jerome P. Lysaught, *You Can Get There from Here: The Orange County/Long Beach Experiment in Improved Patterns of Nursing Education,* The University of Rochester, Rochester, N.Y., 1979, pp. 4–5.
2 Staff papers prepared for the American Hospital Association Advisory Panel on Nurse Shortage, dated November 2, 1978, and February 15, 1979, American Hospital Association, Chicago, 1979 (mimeographed).
3 Jerome P. Lysaught, *An Abstract for Action,* McGraw-Hill Book Company, New York, 1970, p. 131.
4 *Nursing Education and Training: Alternative Federal Approaches,* U.S. Congress, Congressional Budget Office, May 1978, chap. III.
5 Lysaught, *An Abstract for Action,* chap. VI.
6 Jerome P. Lysaught, *From Abstract into Action,* McGraw-Hill Book Company, New York, 1973, chap. VI.
7 Abraham H. Maslow, *Motivation and Personality,* Harper and Row, New York, 1954.

8 F. Herzberg, B. Mausner, and B. B. Snyderman, *The Motivation to Work,* 2d ed., John Wiley & Sons, New York, 1959.

9 Norman E. Amundson, "Labor Relations and the Nursing Leader," in Bonnie Bullough and Vern Bullough (eds.), *Expanding Horizons for Nurses,* Springer Publishing Company, New York, 1977, pp. 204–207.

10 "An Overview of Women in the Workforce," National Commission on Working Women, Center for Women and Work, Washington, D.C., undated newsletter distributed Fall 1978.

11 Lysaught, *From Abstract into Action,* chap. VI, pp. 197–200.

12 Ibid.

13 Ibid.

14 *Report of the American Hospital Association's Advisory Panel on Nurse Shortage,* American Hospital Administration, Chicago, June 6, 1979, p. 5.

15 Bonnie Bullough and Colleen Sparks, "Baccalaureate vs. Associate Degree Nurses: The Care-Cure Dichotomy," in Bullough and Bullough, op. cit., pp. 257–265.

16 Preliminary findings of the Western Interstate Commission on Higher Education Study of state nursing resources and requirements provided by Dr. Eugene Levine, chief, Manpower Analysis and Resources Branch, Division of Nursing, U.S. Department of Health, Education, and Welfare, 1978.

17 Helen K. Grace, "Data Packet: The BSN as Mandatory Threshold to Nursing Practice; Implications for Graduate Nursing Education," University of Illinois, Urbana, October 12, 1978 (mimeographed).

18 *Report of the American Hospital Association's Advisory Panel on Nurse Shortage,* op. cit., p. 10.

19 "JCAH Revises Standards for Hospital Nursing Care," *NLN News* 27(4):5 (April–May 1979).

20 See also Virginia C. Hall, *Statutory Regulation of the Scope of Nursing Practice—A Critical Survey,* The National Joint Practice Commission, Chicago, 1975.

21 Inez G. Hinsvark (director), "The Study of Credentialing in Nursing: A New Approach," *Report of the Committee for the Study of Credentialing in Nursing to the American Nurses' Association,* The University of Wisconsin—Milwaukee, January 1979.

Chapter 7

Summary and Conclusions

Prior to the legal termination of the National Commission for the Study of Nursing and Nursing Education (NCSNN) in 1973, the Commissioners directed the staff to develop a set of protocols for the long-term evaluation of the impact of their attempts to implement the recommendations that had emerged out of the years of study and investigation. From the more than 50 principal recommendations of the Commission's report, *An Abstract for Action,* the staff selected 21 proposals that were critical but that also provided the best guarantees of concomitant variation and temporal relationship—in short, the best assurance that there really existed a cause-effect relationship.

Obviously, it is impossible to argue that there is a simple or singular relationship between any recommendation and the current state of its professional implementation. There are many intervening variables, including such major factors as the state of the economy and the evolving health care delivery structures of our nation, and, in a federal system such as ours, there are bound to be differences in the extent to which any action is taken at the state or regional level. At the same time, many of the recommendations of the National Commission were unique in their concepts and in their implementation: the proposals for joint practice committees, the conceptual framework of episodic and distributive concentrations for education and practice, and the need for a clearinghouse on research findings and generalizations, for example, are clearly traceable to their source in *An Abstract for Action.* What, of course, must be underscored is that the entire process of implementing any—and all —of these recommendations since 1973 lies in the combined efforts of thousands of men and women, nurses and nonnurses, professionals and lay people. This effort, then, is to assess how far the work of reformulation has come and what remains as the unfinished agenda for our largest body of clinical practitioners. Our primary concern is to determine the changes that have occurred rather than to focus on a simplistic cause-effect relationship that might obscure the need for continuing progress and innovation.

In the original planning for the longitudinal examination of the implementation efforts, the National Commission considered the probability of making appropriate surveys at a point some 3 years beyond the lifetime of the NCSNNE. For a variety of reasons, including the obtaining of funds, the development of instruments, the time involved in deriving and analyzing information, and the emergence of related issues such as the 1985 proposal to redefine the entry level for professional nursing, it was determined that the assessment of longitudinal outcomes be extended through 1978—a 5-year period. To adjust for this extension in the period under examination, the statements of anticipated outcomes throughout this summary chapter have been editorially modified as to dates, but no other substantive change has been instituted.

PROPOSALS FOR NURSING ROLES AND FUNCTIONS

The National Commission in 1970 recommended 17 specific proposals for the reorganization and redirection of nursing roles and functions. From this group of proposals, seven were selected as significant benchmarks for the measurement of progress in this area of concern. In 1978, the current study staff undertook the assessment of progress on those recommendations that the Commission considered vital in the development of American nursing. The results are presented and discussed in summary fashion in the following sections.

1   *There will be, in 1978, an operational clearinghouse on nursing research, maintained by a variety of funding agencies and operated under the auspices of the American Nurses' Foundation.*

As strongly as the National Commission urged the necessity for research into the outcomes of nursing intervention and practice, it argued for the utilization of those research findings and their translation into changed behaviors related to client care. To facilitate this process of translating research findings into subsequent clinical applications, it seemed essential that a continuous bibliographic search and retrieval system be developed so that new research reports could be classified, annotated, and arranged to encourage inquiry and utilization. Particularly impressive to the study staff in its investigation of related information systems in other fields were several of the so-called Educational Research Information Centers (ERIC) that were organizing, annotating, and systematizing research findings on such problems in education as the teaching of the handicapped, the utilization of technology, and methods of instruction in the various fields and disciplines.

The development of an annotated bibliographic system capable of rapid and frequent updating would go a long way toward reducing the time gap between the unearthing of new knowledge and its infusion into practice. The American Nurses' Foundation (ANF) was viewed by the Commission as a natural vehicle for receiving both public and private funds and directing them into the establishment and maintenance of a national clearinghouse on nursing research. This organization had been established to encourage nurse researchers and to acquire funds to support small studies and investigations. As a legally independent corporation, it could work cooperatively with all other organizations and elements in nursing to articulate and maintain the proposed clearinghouse and provide the necessary leadership and administrative direction.

Following the distribution of *An Abstract for Action,* the American Nurses' Foundation did develop a formal proposal for the establishment of a clearinghouse on nursing research. This plan was supported by the Council of Nurse Researchers and the Commission on Nursing Research of the American Nurses' Association (ANA) in 1975 and was forwarded to the federal Division of Nursing for funding. In August of that year, the ANF announced that the proposal had not been accepted for funding by the Division, and later the matter was dropped although the Council and the Commission on Nursing Research continued to enunciate their support of the concept.

Site visits to the Division of Nursing and the American Nurses' Foundation in the course of this inquiry indicated that no new initiatives have been undertaken through January of 1979. The Division of Nursing suggested that the function of the clearinghouse could be handled through an extension of the MEDLARS bibliographic service now available through the National Library of Medicine and, furthermore, that any such inquiry system should be operated on a free-for-service basis. There was no indication that support might be provided for the funding of the start-up costs of any viable clearinghouse operation.

The strength of the ERIC systems lay in their annotation and indexing of research entries, in contrast to the basic bibliographic entry form that is used in other retrieval systems. Currently, students and practitioners in nursing have less adequate access to contemporary research in useful, analytic form than do people in many other fields of inquiry. The emergence of new journals in specialty practice fields has helped the situation somewhat, but the lack of a centralized, rapid processing resource facility is continuing to have an adverse effect on the application of knowledge to client care practices.

It is a disappointment to this staff that it must report this recommendation of the National Commission is unrealized to this date and little current activity can be reported to accomplish this end. The need to encourage continuing inquiry into nursing science and practice, the need to disseminate and utilize the findings of that research, and the need to translate them into practice, however, argue that this recommendation be reviewed periodically and that new avenues be examined in the hope of implementation. Recently, the governing structure of the American Nurses' Foundation was reorganized in an effort to expand its activities and enhance its accomplishments and has expressed an interest in reexamining the clearinghouse concept. We suggest to the ANF, to the Council of Nurse Researchers, and to the Commission on Nursing Research that a renewed effort be made to establish a national clearinghouse for studies in nursing and to secure initial funding. The development of a free-for-service operation is not unreasonable, but the system must be in place before users can help to underwrite its continuance.

As this investigation neared its conclusion, however, two fresh developments rekindled the possibility of a systematic approach to the collection and retrieval of nursing research information and the establishment of a national clearinghouse. The Conduct and Utilization of Research in Nursing (CURN) project (a joint effort by the schools of nursing at Michigan and Michigan State Universities) has produced protocols for retrieving, reviewing, and organizing research studies for the purpose of encouraging their transfer into practice. Relatedly, Sigma Theta Tau, the national recognition society for nurse researchers, has begun a directory of researchers as a step toward developing an inquiry and retrieval system. In combination, these efforts bespeak new interests and intentions concerning the codification and utilization of nursing research and its translation into altered practice behaviors. The full extent of their impact must remain to be assessed.

   2   *There will be, in 1978, a statistically significant increase both in the number of foundations making grants in support of nursing research related to practice and in the amounts of money being provided for that purpose.*

In its analysis of the need for strengthened research into nursing practice, the National Commission observed, "Clearly one of the primary reasons for the slow growth of research lies in the lack of financial and institutional support for study activities" [1]. In 1970, almost none of the 100 largest private foundations provided financial support for clinical nursing research. A few supported educational programs and advanced study that involved research components, but this was incidental to the purpose underwritten by the sponsoring agency. The American Nurses' Foundation was established to develop a better understanding of the need for nursing research and to solicit increased support from the private sector in providing funds for investigations. Discussions between this study staff and ANF personnel indicate that some growth took place in the period from 1973 through 1978 in terms of the receipt of private funds, but that these were often earmarked for programmatic purposes that were in the nature of educational or care projects rather than research. In 1979, however, the foundation made eight grants to nurse researchers, and all of these were clinical in nature. An increasing number of corporations and funds have begun to provide research grants and awards to nurses in the specialty practice groups and in advanced clinical settings. In sum, however, any significance is limited to the statistical growth of funds from an almost zero-level base; from the practical standpoint, nursing research still derives sharply limited support from the private sector and most foundations have not included such activity in their designation of priorities.

In the 5-year period concluded in 1978, however, there was a truly significant growth in federal dollars for nursing research resulting in the doubling of funds from approximately $3 million to $6 million.* The rate of growth dropped sharply in 1978, however, and the veto of the Nurse Training Act (NTA) in 1979 casts a large cloud of uncertainty over the future of such allocations. Moreover, state funds for nursing research have been almost solely in the form of some assistance for advanced graduate programs that have a research component. This study staff was unable to document any state funding for nursing research per se. Our surveys of educational institutions and care facilities indicated that some limited support was available to graduate students and practitioners who wished to conduct research, but the amounts from endowments or other sources were quite small and projections for growth were not strongly encouraging.

In short, if the federal allocations for nursing research are reduced or eliminated, the entire support base for examination into nursing practice would collapse. The opportunities to improve patient care and health maintenance through better nursing practice are too important to this nation to permit that debacle. The reliance on federal programs however, places needless limitations on the inquiry process in nursing and tends to inhibit research and researchers through the imposition of extensive bureaucratic requirements. Nursing severely needs an infusion of private funding that could enable more rapid, more discretionary support of small research projects deriving from perceived clinical needs and problems. Quality assurance can be maintained, of course, but the encouragement of research efforts inherently involves greater freedom and choice of alternatives than is currently afforded by governmental approaches alone. There is a great need for "seed" grants and exploration studies that can be mounted with a minimum of delay and overhead costs; again, this need seems particularly attuned to private rather than public support.

It seems essential to this study staff that the reorganized American Nurses' Foundation, the Council of Nurse Researchers, and the Commission on Nursing Research redouble their efforts to educate the private sector on the success of our modest efforts to date in nursing inquiry and to convince foundations, corporations, philanthropic agencies, and nurses themselves of the need to expand our knowledge of nursing science and practice. Certainly, nurses should strive to maintain and expand the levels of federal support for nursing research, but diversified sources of assistance must be developed and maintained. Feedback of findings, accomplishments, and impacts must be an integral part of this effort so that private elements recognize that their contributions are being used effectively and to real purpose. The challenge is great, but the need is greater and the possibilities for good greater still.

Perhaps the most encouraging short-run development in nursing research lies in the commitment of an increased number of colleges and universities to mount

---

*The impact of inflation over this period of time, however, meant that the growth rate in real dollars was considerably less than double.

doctoral programs emphasizing conceptual and clinical research. In the face of limited public and private support for research funding, this would indicate a firm belief in the ability of nursing to demonstrate quality and significance in investigative efforts and, most of all, confidence in the profession's ability to transfer knowledge into improved practice. It may well be that a commitment to the preparation of nurse-doctorates trained in research is a necessary forerunner to the acquisition of monetary support. In the furtherance of the National Commission's plea for an enlarged knowledge base to guide nursing practice, this study staff urges the support of these doctoral training programs by public and private agencies.

3   *There will be, in 1978, an operational National Joint Practice Commission sponsored by the American Medical Association and the American Nurses' Association, this commission to be actively engaged in carrying out the activities proposed by the National Commission for the Study of Nursing and Nursing Education.*

By any measure the National Joint Practice Commission (NJPC) is alive and well—and actively engaged in the activities proposed by the NCSNNE. Composed of 16 members, 8 each from the American Medical Association (AMA) and ANA, the commission has had one full-time director, Dr. William B. Schaffrath, since its inception. In its 5 years of existence, the NJPC has initiated continuing dialogue between nurses and physicians at all levels of interrelationship from national conferences and meetings to local hospital joint committees. It has from time to time issued statements or positions on issues of significance for joint delivery of health care and has engaged in a number of demonstration projects designed to encourage new practitioner relationships between physicians and nurses.

In 1977, the NJPC published *Together: A Casebook of Joint Practices in Primary Care* [2], which documents a number of collaborative approaches to the reformulation of both medical and nursing practice so as to improve the quality of client care through the best utilization of clinical capabilities. In order to facilitate the legal considerations of these evolving patterns, the NJPC commissioned a study on the statutory regulation of the scope of nursing practice which included a careful review of medical and nursing practice acts and examined ways of properly covering the expanded role of the nurse while ensuring the basic integrity of public regulation and client safety [3].

Not all the NJPC activities and recommendations have been greeted with warm approval. Many physicians are distrustful of the clinical care provided by nurse practitioners and clinical specialists; quite a few nurses chafe at the lack of freedom actually accorded them and the degree of control that still obtains in supposedly collaborative practice situations. As compared with the almost complete breakdown in communications that was evident in 1968, however, it is to the credit of the NJPC that there is meaningful dialogue and a closing gap in understanding between these two key groups of health practitioners. As a further measure of the need to continue these efforts at cooperation and collaboration, our surveys of state nurses' associations in 1978 indicated that physicians, in the opinion of the respondents, still held somewhat negative views about an expanded professional role for nursing. The state groups felt a need for better communication and joint planning. (It is significant to point out that specialty practice groups in nursing reported a much more positive reaction by physicians to their extension of clinical roles, thus suggesting the importance of NJPC's insistence on bringing practitioners from the professions together to address their common concerns for patient care and its improvement.)

Another point of controversy in NJPC's effort to broaden the scope of joint practice followed the issuance of its "Statement on Nursing Staffs in Hospitals." In addition to stressing the responsibility of nursing to assume authority and responsibility for the quality of patient care rendered by nurses and for the ethical conduct and professional practices of their staff members, the commission proposed that nursing be accountable to the governing board of the hospital rather than to the administrator. Although this was perceived to be an essential step toward parity with medicine in terms of professional influence on decision making, the American Hospital Association Board of Trustees and Council on Professional Services expressed their concerns over this departure from traditional organizational arrangements in hospitals in which nursing service reports to the administrator. Efforts are now under way to discuss these and other concerns related to NJPC concepts of nurse staffing in an emergent hospital care system [4].

There is little disagreement with the viewpoint that the NJPC has served as a catalyst and as a leader in the reexamination of nurse-physician relations. It may be that the scope of discussions will more frequently move from the dyadic relations of these two professions to a three-cornered relationship that includes the administrators of health care facilities. If so, the NJPC has already anticipated many of the most substantive problems and in its statements on joint practice in primary care and joint practice in hospitals has pointed the way to improving the welfare of the patient by involving medicine, nursing, and administration in the decision-making process. It is hoped that the Commission will resolve those issues that it has identified and examined. Meanwhile, its objectivity and interdisciplinary membership ensures that its recommendations will be given thoughtful consideration even by those who are disturbed by its somewhat iconoclastic approach to the customary arrangements for providing health care.

4   *There will be, in 1978, joint practice committees in each state, involved in improving the delivery of health care through better nurse-physician practice patterns.*

The staff of the National Commission aimed in 1973 at the universal spread of statewide counterpart groups to the National Joint Practice Committee, but there were many persons at the state level who were very pessimistic that any concrete arrangements for interprofessional planning and discussion could be effected or continued over a prolonged period. In 1978, our present study staff identified 41 states in which joint practice committees were operational and several additional states in which discussions about the feasibility of such a group is under way.

If our best hopes have not been realized, there is a considerable amount of accomplishment to record. These state committees have been involved in the definition of collaborative practice, the rewriting of state practice acts, and the development of statements of opinion for release by state attorneys general speaking to the expanding role of the nurse and the new relationships of delegation and supervision between the two practitioner groups. Many of these statewide joint practice committees were involved in the amendment or rewriting of nurse practice acts in no less than 39 separate jurisdictions since 1973. In almost every instance, the changed provisions of those statutes were designed to enlarge the scope of nursing practice and to define the nursing role in less restrictive terms.

In the spring of 1978, the National Joint Practice Commission surveyed its state counterpart committees in order to learn of current activities and areas of concern. Among the highlights revealed in the returns are these: the encouragement of local joint practice committees in institutions for health care delivery, the encouragement of primary nursing in hospital settings as well as in distributive care facilities, the formulation of statewide policies and scope of practice statements for nurse practitioners and clinical specialists, and the extension of hospital privileges to nonemployee nurse practitioners [5]. Typically, there was considerable variance among the reporting states on the progress achieved in the different areas, but there is no gainsaying that even the discussion of these matters would not have taken place a decade ago, nor would it be likely to be taking place today in the absence of the national and statewide joint practice groups.

It was an article of faith with the National Commission for the Study of Nursing and Nursing Education that nurses and physicians could and would work collaboratively when the primary point at issue was the improvement of client care. The joint practice committees have borne out this faith, and in the next round of development —at the local, institutional level—we anticipate that understanding and cooperation will continue to increase, with concomitant benefits to the delivery of care.

5 *There will be, in 1978, a statistically significant shift in the allocation of nursing manpower with a major increase in the numbers and percentages of nurse practitioners in the area of distributive care.*

Traditionally, the bulk of the practitioner force in nursing could be found in the hospital setting, whereas most analyses of our health care requirements agree that the majority of our problems at any given time relate to health maintenance and minor illness that have nothing to do with the "heavy" apparatus and technology of our episodic treatment centers. Although the percentage of nurses employed in 1978 (approximately 89 percent) was still heavily weighted toward the hospital, this figure masks a great deal of change that has occurred over the last 5 years. First of all, an increasing number of medical centers, teaching hospitals, and community hospitals have expanded significantly into the development of health maintenance organizations, ambulatory and outpatient clinics, and the general provision of nonacute care. Second, there has been pronounced growth within clinical fields of nursing toward the enlargement of the scope of practice to include distributive care as well as episodic treatment. The Nurses' Association of the American College of Obstetricians and Gynecologists, for example, has emphasized new roles in family planning, prenatal and postnatal care and counseling, human sexuality, and total family involvement in care and delivery. Third, there has been a recognizable redirection of nursing roles in the traditional distributive areas of public health, school nursing, and occupational health toward more clinical involvement and expanded practice. Thus, the number of nurses employed in episodic agencies and facilities is still commanding, but the greatest proportional shift has been toward the distributive areas of nursing; the nurses' numbers have increased, and, more important, their functions have become far more clinical and far less administrative and clerical.

These observations are verified by our survey of state nurses' associations. In 1978, 75 percent of the states reported growth in the utilization of nurses for clinical distributive care; 63 percent of the states reported that this growth was pronounced in their areas. The importance of these figures goes far beyond the findings. In any clinical discipline, it is a truism that practice generally precedes educational change. Role change first takes place in the client setting and then is molded into the academic curriculum once it has been proven to be effective and efficient. In 1968, preparatory programs in nursing were essentially aimed at producing episodic clinicians. With the growth of distributive practice, it is highly significant that 46 percent of all baccalaureate institutions included in our national survey offered clinical concentrations in both episodic and distributive care and another 32 percent offered a choice of clinical concentrations using other descriptive terminology. Associate degree programs have been less prone to change their curricula; only 50 percent offer some kind of clinical concentration that might include nonepisodic dimensions. Surprisingly 44 percent of the reporting hospital schools of nursing have indicated the inclusion of clinical choices in episodic and distributive care—undoubtedly reacting to the point that hospitals are no longer "cure" institutions alone, but are putting heavy emphasis on health maintenance and nonacute care facilities.

There is evidence of a shift in nursing roles and positions toward greater commitment to distributive care, but it is too early to tell how well we are equipped to meet the emerging demands for a full range of health services. One estimate by the Department of Health, Education, and Welfare (HEW) indicates that 20 million Americans will be enrolled in health maintenance organizations by the end of 1980. In all likelihood, nursing will be quite capable of filling the distributive care roles required for that level of demand. Whether, however, there would be sufficient practitioners to respond to greater needs—if, for example, there were national health insurance or even a tremendous surge of health maintenance coverage by private insurers and third-party payers—is quite doubtful.

There has been in most areas of the country a significant shift toward increased nursing involvement in the practice of distributive care. With the impact of new nurse practice acts, the expansion of roles in these fields will increase. The curricula of nursing schools are being rearranged in the light of these developments. The unknown element is the rate of growth of demand; for the time being, this would seem to be within the limits of nursing response, but manpower planners must monitor developments in the light of diversified nursing practice.

6   *There will be, in 1978, a statistically significant upward shift in the proportion of time spent by nurses in all health care facilities in direct client contact and a*

statistically significant downward shift in the utilization of nurses for supervisory and administrative functions within all health care facilities.

One of the vexing concerns of the National Commission from its inception lay in the traditional patterns for nursing service in American hospitals and other care facilities. Promotion to the next higher levels in nursing hierarchies inevitably led away from patient care and into administrative and organizational concerns that were essentially institutional rather than clinical matters. Nurse administrators were functioning as hospital middle managers rather than as leaders in the enhancement of patient care through clinical nursing intervention. This, of course, was true as a generalization, but we saw such singular exceptions that we argued for a redirection of the entire structure of nursing roles so that reward, recognition, and promotion should be built around patient care and that excellence in clinical practice, rather than institutional administration, should become the primary criterion for advancement.

In 1978, this study staff surveyed 183 hospitals across the country to determine whether they perceived any shift in the proportions of time devoted to clinical concerns and institutional matters. The response was encouraging, but indicated that much more change is needed. Slightly more than 61 percent of the directors of nursing service reported a significant upward shift in the emphasis on clinical excellence for reward, recognition, and promotion. A disturbing element, however, lies in the frequency with which the remaining directors reported that efforts to move in this direction were forestalled by collective bargaining agreements that insist upon seniority as the primary basis for any promotion in nursing service.

Three out of every four hospitals reported that supervisory nurses are now expected to be more clinically competent than staff nurses and to function as clinical leaders in patient care. This is in marked contrast to our findings in 1970, which indicated that supervisory nurses then spent, on average, about 7 percent of their time in direct patient care with the vast majority of their work being devoted to institutional concerns and administrative requirements. In 1978, almost three-quarters of the reporting institutions indicated that all nursing service personnel were spending more time in clinical functions than was the case in 1973, and an increasing number of institutions are hiring nurse practitioners and clinical specialists to extend the scope of nursing service within their facilities. Changing assignment patterns throughout our health care system indicate that nurses are increasing patient contact and divesting themselves of nonnursing functions.

Having said that much, the darker side of the picture emerges. Only about 25 percent of the hospitals have actually budgeted positions for nurse practitioners or clinical specialists, and approximately 33 percent have designated one or more positions for certified nurse practitioners. Essentially, these constraints appear to be budgetary and financial. This is further borne out by the Whyte study on the effects of certification for advanced practice, which found that there was little economic reward attached to such recognition—though role enlargement and increased responsibility did take place in most instances [6].

In effect, it would appear that we are developing a new and different look to the clinical practice of hospital nursing, but we are still using traditional models for budgeting and economic allocation. This realization, in part, led the American Hospital Association's Advisory Panel on the Nurse Shortage to recommend that a research and development group look into the practical economics of new staffing patterns and role expectations to see if there are not sound financial reasons, as well as clinical motivations, to change from our present configurations [7]. The National Joint Practice Committee, through a grant from the W. K. Kellogg Foundation, is currently exploring the enhancement of patient care through a combination of primary nursing, joint practice and collaboration, and the utilization of all-R.N. staffs in the clinical areas under study [8].

It is clearly evident that reorganization of roles in nursing service is taking place and that clinical practice is becoming a much greater force than it was in 1970 or 1973, but it is essential that we develop hard data and documentation on the clinical *and* economic outcomes of primary nursing, differentiated staffing, and advanced clinical practice—as well as many other experimental elements that are being tested in individual institutions across the country. Traditional staffing concepts are hard to bend or break, and the current pressures for budgetary restraint maximize the forces that fear the impact of change.* Unfortunately, the status quo with all its problems, may be more attractive to some administrators and directors of nursing service than the uncertainty of new patterns for staffing, utilization, and compensation. To convince them—and many other health planners and government functionaries—this study staff believes we need the outcomes of the NJPC projects and the documented results proposed by the American Hospital Association (AHA) advisory committee to guide us along.

More experimentation is needed in nurse staffing for health care facilities, but any research or demonstration project funded by public agencies or private foundations should be required to maintain evaluative records on both clinical outcomes and economic impact. Further progress toward better utilization of nursing service will be deterred unless more substantive data are available to those who must bear the responsibility for decision making.

7   *There will be, in 1978, a statistically significant upward shift in the number of institutions offering joint appointments in education and service and in the number of individual faculty members who are actively engaged in the practice of nursing in addition to teaching.*

In 1970, there were only a handful of institutions that offered joint appointments in education and service. This was a source of concern not only to the Commission, but also to many of our advisory groups, which felt that more faculty should be excellent practitioners, that fine clinicians should be responsible, in part, for the development of students, and that the profession of nursing would be the stronger for a rapprochement between these two arms of a single entity. Accord-

---

*The growing phenomena of nurse pools and registries, with higher attendants costs, may force changes upon administrators, however, in order to contain expenditures.

ingly, the Commission encouraged the concept of a unification style for nursing education and service which would bring these bodies under one roof, not unlike the model of the medical school that combines teaching and practice in a blend of professional development. A number of merged programs in nursing appeared, Rush University and the University of Rochester among them, with the direction of education and service lodged in one office or position. Nevertheless, this could be a viable pattern at the present only for schools of nursing affiliated with major health care centers or teaching hospitals.

As an interim or alternative measure to a full unification model, the Commission urged the greater use of joint appointments and responsibilities shared between educational and service institutions. In 1978, our study staff was able to document a significant growth in such arrangements, although they are, for the most part, found in baccalaureate and higher degree programs, on the one hand, and university hospitals and Veterans Administration hospitals on the other. Sixty-five percent of the baccalaureate institutions now offer joint appointments and encourage their faculty to be involved in clinical care on an extended basis.* Associate degree programs are far less likely to have such arrangements; only 20 percent of our respondents reported having joint appointments. Less than 6 percent of the hospital schools of nursing utilized this concept. At the same time, however, among service institutions, community hospitals reported that less than 30 percent of their facilities appointed educators to positions of extended commitment to patient care. By the sheer force of numbers, then, the percentage of all hospitals reporting ran at 28 percent utilizing joint appointments, but with 75 percent of the university hospitals and 80 percent of the Veterans Administration hospitals reporting such arrangements.

There have been significant increases in the effort to bring nursing education and service back into a collaborative and interdependent relationship. There is a continuing need, however, to diffuse this movement and to encourage many more educational institutions and care facilities to explore the opportunities to enhance both teaching and clinical practice. Many of the efforts to expand roles, provide primary nursing, and develop advanced clinical practitioners will stand or fall upon the basic agreement between nurse educators and care providers to provide mutual support and committed effort to enlarge the scope of their professional perspectives. A start has been made, but nurse organizations and individuals face great challenges in bringing these concepts into a position where they are seen as normative rather than as exceptional patterns of behavior.

PROPOSALS FOR NURSING EDUCATION

In 1970, the National Commission for the Study of Nursing and Nursing Education advanced 22 recommendations for the improvement and repatterning of nursing

---

*This figure, of course, may be overly positive in the sense that most baccalaureate institutions still have only a small percentage of their faculty involved in joint appointments. The direction and rate of movement are, however, most encouraging.

education. Many of these avowedly were simply updated versions of proposals for nursing education that went back many years to the earlier studies of the profession. Some of these proposals, however, were unique to the findings of the investigative work that led to *An Abstract for Action.* The study staff, in 1973, selected seven of these recommendations as evaluative benchmarks for consideration in any longitudinal examination of the impact of the Commission's work. Those proposals are presented here.

1 *There will be, in 1978, a designated interdisciplinary planning committee in each state charged with general responsibility for coordination of nursing education.*

In *An Abstract for Action,* the National Commission noted that there had been numerous state studies of nursing needs and educational requirements, but that few of these efforts had been crowned with success and extensive implementation. To provide better direction to educational planning and to ensure wider acceptance of the recommendations that might proceed from such efforts, the National Commission proposed the concept of statewide master planning committees that would be interdisciplinary in nature and would be charged with the responsibility for planning an articulated pattern of collegiate education in nursing, including advanced levels, so that sufficient numbers of properly prepared nurses would be available to meet the expanded and differentiated needs of a changing health care delivery system. This charge would include the development of increased cooperation between educational institutions and health care facilities in the planning of educational programs and, particularly, the provision of clinical experience, the articulation of lower- and upper-division programs to facilitate career mobility and individual access to advanced levels of preparatory training, and the most effective utilization of resources so that a system for statewide education emerged that would be attuned to the health care needs of the people.

Originally, the study staff of the National Commission worked with nine target states to establish such master planning committees; after several false starts, it was recognized that states, like persons, possess unique characteristics and that the composition, establishment, location, and workings of each master planning committee must reflect the "personality" of the jurisdiction they sought to guide. Out of the refined efforts of the successful planning bodies, more detailed suggestions for procedures and approaches emerged. In 1978, this study staff surveyed the state nurses' associations to determine the current status of statewide master planning and determined that 32 states (63 percent) have designated bodies serving in this capacity. In most states without master planning committees, there are agencies within the state board of higher education which provide for some of the functions proposed by the National Commission, but the results are quite variable—and sometimes unpredictable.

In at least three of the states that reported no master planning committee, there are activities under way and proposals drafted to initiate such bodies, but many of the states feel that there is simply insufficient interest or perceived need at the present time to inspire work in this direction.

There should be considerable satisfaction over the establishment and success of so many of these master planning committees. The problems of nonarticulation and of nonsystematic planning for varied levels and specialties in nursing education and practice, however, are too compelling to be neglected. Perhaps the "lack of interest" reported in some 13 states is more a reflection of our inability to present the problems clearly and forcefully. So long as noncollegiate and collegiate programs turn out nurses, so long as articulation between lower- and upper-division programs is left to chance, and so long as the primary concern of planners and administrators is preparatory programs rather than a progressive flow of nursing students along identifiable paths to advanced clinical levels, then there are problems in the planning of nursing education which require solution.

It is essential not only that more statewide master planning committees be established for those states that lack them, but also that some periodic effort be made to reexamine proposed master plans and to update them from time to time based on new patterns for both education and practice. Much has been done, and well done, but planning is a continuing process that must not be neglected or allowed to become disfunctional through obsolescence.

   2   *There will be, in 1978, a significant increase in joint planning between hospitals schools and colleges prior to the termination of diploma programs.*

In 1970, of course, the National Commission proposed the reorganization of all nursing education within the mainstream of our collegiate patterns for higher education. Some analysts of health economics predicted that hospital schools of nursing would essentially disappear by 1980 without any other intervention than that of cost. The NCSNNE and its staff were not so persuaded. The issue of hospital schools had long been fraught with emotionalism, anger, and extremism. Moreover, without joint discussion and planning, any changes would likely be chaotic and arbitrary— with the burden of impact falling on the students, who were the most vulnerable individuals in the battle of institutional determinism.

Accordingly, the Commission urged the transition of nursing education into the collegiate system, but urged that no program close—or any open—until there had been adequate planning and provision of alternatives to ensure an orderly change process. Between the start of the Commission's investigation and its close in 1973, the number of hospital schools of nursing was reduced almost one-third. Between 1973 and 1978, this group of institutions was reduced by another 26 percent. Meanwhile, collegiate programs have grown in number and proportion so that they now represent 80 percent of all admissions to preparatory nursing programs.

Although the Commission and its staff worked arduously to aid in this transitional process, it was never our thought that the reduction of diploma programs would be a valid benchmark for the evaluation of our implementation efforts. Too many other variables were at work for anyone to partial out the influence of one factor. On the other hand, the Commission, more than any other single agency, sought to work with the Council of Diploma Programs and the Assembly of Hospital Schools of Nursing to bring data and planning to bear on the future of nursing graduates as well as that of their institutions and to examine ways in which positive aspects of new patterns for nursing education might be fostered.

Out of this planning, some hospital schools made the commitment to become collegiate institutions in their own right and succeeded in this endeavor. More hospital schools made the decision to close, but only through negotiations with collegiate programs that strengthened cooperative ties and enhanced the clinical learning opportunities for the students considerably. Many hospital schools remain in operation, and some are vociferous in their determination to continue for all time to come. In our survey of a striated sample of educational institutions for nursing, we asked the respondents whether they were currently engaged in interinstitutional planning to enhance the articulation of curricula and the mobility of students. Fifty percent of the reporting hospital schools of nursing indicated that they were actively involved in such discussions. To this study staff, this is a measure of the National Commission's success in getting disparate elements of nursing education to come together and to seek common ground and orderly processes for transition. Without communication and without understanding no change is possible.

We are not sanguine about the current situation. More than 340 hospital schools of nursing exist, and, for the most part, these are larger, stronger, more militant than those that have closed their doors. Incredibly enough, since 1973, two new hospital schools of nursing have opened in the face of recommendations going back to 1923 that these institutions phase out of existence! But since 1973 there has been no evidence of leadership among the national organizations for nursing to effect a final solution to the bifurcated system of preparatory education that has had such a sorry impact on the profession and on the careers of hundreds of thousands of nurses.

Either the National League for Nursing (NLN), the currently designated body for accreditation of programs for nursing education, or the newly proposed Nurse Credentialing Center (NCC) must take responsibility for ending the divisive routes of entry into nursing, which make it the only body of its size and professional protestations that maintains a noncollegiate track alongside its collegiate track through higher education. The discussion and planning phase must be followed by decision and action. National leadership is required. It should not be necessary to add that, if and when the NLN or the NCC resolves to move on this matter, it should have the support of all other professional groups that claim to speak for nurses and nursing.

3   *There will be, in 1978, a significant increase in the articulation between 2- and 4-year institutions with a statistically significant increase in the number of baccalaureate institutions that offer upper-division programs in anticipation of enrolling graduates of A.D.N. programs.*

Our survey of educational institutions indicates that there has been a significant increase in the dialogue of articulation between upper- and lower-division programs. Sixty-one percent of the baccalaureate programs and 56 percent of the associate degree programs reported that they were involved in interinstitutional planning for increased mobility and transfer. This is most encouraging, but it must also be pointed out that they reported a variety of problems in their search for better linkages. The time involved in joint planning and the costs involved in released time, meeting expenses, and travel expenses are not inconsiderable even when institutions are geographically near. The reality of differences between institutional policies is also a matter of grave concern. Finally, there are matters of nursing politics that impede the progress of articulation. If, for example, many of the baccalaureate faculty view associate degree nurses as technicians and not as beginning professionals, then the best intentions of a joint planning committee may be doomed. Nevertheless, in 1978, no less than 78 percent of the reporting baccalaureate programs indicate that they have a systematic plan for the matriculation of R.N.'s into their program—though many added that such positions are necessarily limited by the demands of their institution's own students for admission to the nursing sequence.

Because most baccalaureate programs in 1970 were of the *generic* variety—that is, essentially 2 years of arts and science followed by 2 years of nursing education —there was always a discomforting lack of fit between these curricular expectations and the experiential background that R.N.'s from hospital and associate degree programs presented upon request for admission. To maintain the integrity of the generic programs and still serve the need for career mobility and access, the National Commission urged the establishment of upper-division programs in baccalaureate nursing that would be specifically planned for the graduate of a lower-division R.N. program. The person completing such a program would, on balance, have achieved similar competencies to those of the generic graduate, but would have arrived at them by a different—not inferior—route. It was the Commission's belief that large institutions might have operational programs of both kinds, generic and upper-division, and that other institutions might elect one or the other. A large demonstration project, the Orange County/Long Beach Consortium for Nursing Education, developed a cooperative arrangement that included five community colleges, two state university campuses, and a medical center with a school of medicine. Aided by a grant from the W. K. Kellogg Foundation, a series of behavioral competencies and objectives were developed and linked in such fashion that the output of one level was the defined input for the next successive level [9]. Similar statements of competencies were developed through the Southern Regional Education Board (SREB) Nursing Curriculum Project [10].

With the evidence that lower/upper-division articulation can and does work, some 45 programs were operational by the end of 1978, and more are projected in the months ahead, with the first national conference on research into such educational programs slated for early 1980. Nevertheless, some leaders in nursing education are unconvinced that these articulated programs provide the quality of generic programs, and there have been strong feelings aroused that accreditation visits and decisions on the upper-division type programs made by "traditionalists" have been unduly harsh and negative. This opposition prompted a strenuous and successful effort to place the Council on Baccalaureate and Higher Degree programs of the National League for Nursing on record as supporting and promoting quality in nontraditional nursing programs.

With the impetus of the 1985 proposal and the growing concern over bolstering enrollments in baccalaureate programs of all descriptions, it is very likely that the concept of articulation between 2- and 4-year institutions will soon be satisfactorily resolved. There is already evidence that the system can work and can turn out able professionals with enlarged clinical knowledge and skills. The beginning efforts should be expanded so that adequate openings exist in programs appropriate to the needs of registered nurses.

4   *There will be, in 1978, a significant increase in the number of area or regional consortia for nursing education with shared facility, faculty, and resources.*

In 1970, the National Commission urged that smaller preparatory programs for nursing be closed and that larger programs be expanded to provide the same number of positions and graduates but with an economy of resources and a better redistribution of human and capital investment. As one way of achieving this, the Commission cited the example of the Spokane consortium for nursing education, which actually united a number of small programs into one administrative entity, and the Orange County/Long Beach Consortium, which, through joint planning, effected a division of effort and a commitment to specializations that would eliminate overlap and redundancy. The success of these two approaches argued forcefully for their adoption in other localities. Moreover, the Southern Regional Educational Board had long taken leadership in such areas as planning for graduate nursing education in the South to prevent unreasonable growth and competition beyond the needs and resources of the region.

Since 1973, the number of preparatory programs in nursing has remained relatively stable, the greatest redistribution being the reduction in hospital schools of nursing and the growth of collegiate programs. This has been accompanied by a slow rate of growth in the number of admissions per program, but the situation in 1978 ought to be a matter of concern. Nationally, we admit, on average, 84 students per program per year. Baccalaureate institutions have the highest class average, with 106 students. Associate degree programs admit an average of 83, and hospital schools of nursing average 61 admissions. It would seem that programs that consistently enroll less than 50 students per class—unless they are avowedly experimental in nature—should seriously consider the possibility of enlargement, merger, or termination in order to assure a more economical allocation of resources.

No significant increase has taken place in the number of regional consortia for nursing education, in part, of course, because of institutional reluctance to lose identity or diminish control, but also because of funding problems. It may be that statewide master planning committees and boards of higher education will have to play a leadership role in determining the minimum size and resources for nursing programs within their jurisdictions. The National Commission opted for enlightened self-interest, and this has failed to materialize as an answer.

5   *There will be, in 1978, no less than three completed regional or area studies of the nursing curriculum with proposals for universals or core studies, alternatives or specializations, and sequential approaches to articulation.*

In 1978, this study staff examined carefully the experiences and the publications of two major curriculum development projects both of which were supported substantially by the W. K. Kellogg Foundation. The Southern Regional Educational Board through its Nursing Curriculum Project has developed a series of competencies for the graduates of associate degree, baccalaureate, and graduate programs in nursing. The Orange County/Long Beach Consortium has done essentially the same thing and has employed these behavioral descriptions as the exit and entry levels for the institutional curricula throughout the region. Although they were not mobilized in the sense of the studies mentioned above, a number of institutions and statewide planning groups have examined curricular articulation and planned for career mobility in such ways as to justify our staff's conclusion that this objective has been fairly achieved.

Three observations, however, on the experience of these curriculum planners seem pertinent based on our site visits, interviews, and review of materials. First, the probing study of curriculum and articulation becomes more complex than any of the Commission staff thought when they proposed this activity in 1970. The SREB Nursing Curriculum Project, for example, felt it necessary to develop companion projects in nontraditional studies, faculty development in clinical care, evaluation of student clinical practice, and a number of other areas. Many of these issues had to be explored in the Orange County/Long Beach studies as well. The widening nature of these concerns requires tremendous commitments of time and effort on the part of those involved—and a willingness to be stern self-critics.

A second observation is that there has been some ripple effect, but not nearly the amount of contagion that the National Commission might have expected in 1973. One example of success is the interaction between the Orange County/Long Beach development and the New Mexico statewide plan for articulated nursing education throughout that state. The basic elements of the California consortium have been utilized extensively, with appropriate modifications of the New Mexico assessment of needs and resources. Undoubtedly, many institutions have used the SREB or California materials in their internal planning. What is not obvious is that other regional bodies, such as the New England or Western Interstate associations for nursing education, have attempted to utilize and adapt these approaches on a concerted basis. No organization, in short, has assumed the leadership role in implementing the generalizations from these studies in regions outside the point of origin. It would seem that more of the various regional associations might develop cooperative approaches to the utilization of materials and resources once they have been initiated anywhere in the country. The issue, of course, is broader than the matter of curricular study, but this could be a valuable starting point.

The third observation is that tradition and the status quo are not easily overcome in the academic setting. One writer on higher education has remarked that college faculty are the most liberal people in the world on every issue except academics, and that there they become the most conservative people in the world. Despite the long and thoughtful process that led to the development of the competencies and behaviors at the various levels or stages of these articulated plans, many nurse educators blithely dismiss the entire concept because they see any alternative to traditional curricular arrangements as a dilution or corruption of educational integrity. Out of many, many discussions, site visits, conferences, and workshops, this study staff is convinced that curricular change must be constantly championed and that its advocates must be committed realists. Innovation is always uncomfortable —even for its proponents. Academic innovation is peculiarly abrasive, it would appear. Institutions and individuals who adopt the new curricular patterns will find themselves under great pressure to conform for the next several years. With perseverance, however, we can look for enhanced career mobility and individual access throughout the structure of nursing education because of their initiatives.

   6   *There will be, in 1978, a significant increase in the number of programs at both 2-year and 4-year institutions which offer a concentration in episodic and/or distributive care.*

   In 1970, the National Commission coined the terms *episodic* and *distributive care* to distinguish two general positions in a conceptual framework that included nursing behaviors, client condition, and environmental settings. Our purpose in doing this was to emphasize that much of the traditional curriculum and instructional content in nursing was built, consciously or not, around the hospital-medical service model for practice—and to point out that there were whole other worlds of need for nursing care, in health maintenance, mild unwellness, and chronic illness, which were not being touched. Perhaps no other proposal of the Commission touched off a greater debate.

   Once the initial flurry of excitment passed, however, many nurse educators did reexamine the curricular arrangements of their programs and were surprised to find that *illness* dominated many of the assumptions and premises and that *wellness* was hardly touched upon. In 1978, our study staff reviewed survey returns from a striated sample of all preparatory programs in nursing education and were gratified to find that 37 percent of all the respondents offered clinical concentrations in episodic or distributive care; among baccalaureate institutions the figure was 46 percent. Still more encouraging was the fact that another 29 percent of all preparatory programs offered clinical concentrations based on conceptual schemes other than episodic/distributive. In total, then, two-thirds of the reporting institutions had adopted some form of clinical concentration that modified the curriculum that had existed in 1970.

   It is our conclusion that the curricular changes recorded in this survey justify our assertion of significance. The NCSNNE believed that there was—and is—a distinct value to the theoretical framework of episodic and distributive care, but we were far more concerned about the implicit and unexamined characteristics of the nursing curriculum we found in 1970. Innovation, variety, and experimentation are the soul of curricular improvement; the data of 1978 indicated that a considerable unfreezing had taken place in nursing education; and we have no quarrel with those individuals and institutions that have opted for conceptual schemes other than our own. Indeed, any curricular orthodoxy could become oppressive, and we need a variety of competing viewpoints to elicit the best formulations of educational thought.

7   *There will be, in 1978, a significant increase in the number of states that have designated agencies and master plans for the offering of continuing education for nurses and a significant increase in the number and percentage of nurses participating in continuing education.*

If any of the estimates of the National Commission staff was understated, it surely must have been this statement about continuing education. Nine states have already passed mandatory continuing legislation for nursing, and others are very close to adopting such measures. Even where continuing education is voluntary, the emphasis placed on its importance by nursing organizations, specialty practice groups, and health care facilities has greatly increased offerings and registrations.

The American Nurses' Association Council on Continuing Education has played an active role in formulating a nationwide accreditation effort in which state nurses' associations, specialty practice groups, and educational institutions have participated. Statewide and regional efforts have begun to emerge, and many more collegiate institutions have opened departments or divisions of continuing education based on the demand for increased learning opportunities.

It may seem the nadir of negativism to express concern over what is generally so bright a picture, but our site visits and discussions with nurse associations and continuing education directors cause us to pass on some of their concerns because there are worrisome signs in the midst of so much that is positive. There are considerable problems and costs attached to the record-keeping procedures in those states that have mandatory requirements for continuing education. Likewise, differences in requirements for continuing education among the states could lead to increased difficulties for reciprocal recognition or endorsement. Finally, there is the inherent regression to the bureaucratic mean for those groups that become the accreditors of continuing education even though they may not function as either providers or consumers. By this, we simply mean that it is easier to specify such requirements as contact hours, facilities, and reporting methods than it is to deal with content, learning, and significance. It will be a challenge to the Council on Continuing Education and all the other concerned groups to see that the great promise of these developments is not lost in a welter of procedures and paperwork.

PROPOSALS FOR NURSING CAREERS

In 1970, the National Commission sought to end the perennial concern for the nursing "shortage" by developing the concept of career perspectives within the profession. The supposed shortage of nurses could be solved within a very short period of time if we would only address the problem of retention—or the lack thereof —in nursing. Almost half of all the graduate registered nurses in the United States are totally inactive, if we include those who have dropped their license to practice. The reasons can be documented and verified. They include the fact that the basic reward systems—economic, social, and psychological—for nursing are simply insufficient to motivate people over long periods of time. Those people who aspire to leadership and commitment find they are inevitably drawn away from clinical prac-

tice. For too long a time, there has been no career in patient care. To redress these
flaws and to develop career patterns that could retain nurses in their profession, the
National Commission proposed 19 recommendations. Of those, seven are treated
here as an evaluation of longitudinal outcomes related to Commission proposals.

1   *There will be, in 1978, a statistically significant increase in the number of
nurses involved in comprehensive and regional planning and a significant increase in
the percentage of such bodies having nurse members.*

It is a simple truism that one characteristic of a *professional* is the relatively
large scope society grants to that person's decision making and judgment. By this
standard, however, it would have been difficult to perceive nursing as a profession
a decade ago. Nurses simply were not involved in the decision-making processes
related to health care delivery—even as to their own role in carrying out policies
adopted by others. As the National Commission examined the composition of
planning and policy groups in 1968, it was obvious that nurses were not adequately
represented: sometimes they were wholly excluded; sometimes there was tokenism
through the inclusion of one or two individuals, who found it most difficult to press
their viewpoints.

To develop a career perspective for nursing, the National Commission argued
that nurses must become principals to the planning and policy decisions related to
health care and that their contributions to the enhancement of client care would
essentially be equal to their professional involvement in the decision-making process.
To paraphrase an observation by Goethe, if you treat nurses as they are, they will
remain that way, but if you treat them as they could be, they will become that way.
Our conviction was that nurses could help improve planning and policies in 1968,
but could improve them even more in the years to come through continued participation in the fact-finding and negotiation processes.

We feel this has certainly been the case. Beginning with their contributions to
the statewide master planning committees and the joint practice committees, nurses
have become more and more involved in decisions on the emergent health care
delivery system. In 1978, 37 state nurses' associations (73 percent) reported that
nurses in their states have been effectively involved in health planning within the
state and have given leadership to the Health Service Agencies and other mechanisms for determining plans and policies. The remaining 14 states reported that
nurses were serving on planning and development committees, but that there were
still limitations on their ability to contribute. It is clear, however, that nurses are
far more involved than they were in 1968 and 1973, and their involvement is adding
a new dimension to our consideration of client needs and conditions.

2   *There will be, in 1978, a statistically significant alteration in the organizational apportionment of nursing salaries, with significant increases being provided to
clinical nurses and master nurse clinicians in comparison with supervisory nurses.*

Nursing salaries have increased rapidly since 1973, but the impact of inflation
reduces the real gain to a very moderate increase of, perhaps 12 to 15 percent.

Moreover, there is evidence that registered nurses have lost ground in comparison with other health workers. Licensed practical nurses, for example, actually enjoyed a faster rate of increase than did registered nurses, and the current projections are for that trend to continue to occur. In our survey of state nursing associations, there are indications of regional variations of significant proportions in nursing salaries. Fifteen states (30 percent) reported that salary increments over the past 3 years have been adequate or very adequate; more than two-thirds of the states, however, feel that salary increases have been inadequate for their nurses. The true state of affairs, of course, is difficult to determine.

On balance, there has certainly not been the overall gain in nursing salaries, based on and built around patient care, that the National Commission had hoped to see in 1978. In part, this has occurred because within the national economy, the erosion of inflation has reduced the true growth of earnings by as much as two-thirds. In this, of course, nursing suffers along with every other occupational and professional group and cannot hope to be made singularly immune from a societal plague. At the same time, however, nursing seemingly has failed to maintain the meager advantages that it enjoyed relative to other health occupations. This situation calls for serious examination and redress if we are ever to retain our best nurses in a career commitment to patient care.

There is greater evidence than in 1973, however, of higher differentiation in nursing salaries. The mean reported full-time salary for a clinical nurse specialist in 1978 was approximately 42 percent greater than the full-time salary reported for a staff nurse. This growth in economic rewards centered around patient care is certainly in the direction advocated by the National Commission and represents a significant gradation that could have a real impact on retention and on the hygiene factors associated with nursing. Unfortunately, our national survey of hospitals indicated that only about 37 percent of those institutions have adopted salary structures with incremental increases for clinical nurses specialists and clinical practitioners. Essentially this would seem to be a budgetary and economic constraint, which is consistent with the findings of Whyte that critical-care nurses who sought and achieved certification of their own volition seldom received salary increases for this effort [11]. Indeed, some individuals reported that administrators reacted in a negative way to their certification, as if it were a ploy directed at forcing a salary increase.

The beginnings of a differentiated salary scale that pays more for nurses to stay in patient care than to administer the institution is just beginning to emerge. If more care facilities define levels of advanced clinical competency and develop graduated salaries that represent a true evaluation of social worth and contribution to patient care, then we will be well on our way to the development of a career perspective in nursing and to the end of the interminable contemplation of nurse shortages.

In 1970 and 1973, the National Commission was chided by some advocates of economic and general welfare programs in nursing because it did not endorse the concept of collective bargaining for nurses. The Commissioners felt that there were preferable professional approaches to the development of an adequate and career minded pattern of compensation. This study staff still endorses that approach, but with a growing feeling of urgency that health administrators, economists, planners, and third-party payers must reexamine their basic premises regarding nursing and join with that profession to establish not only adequate entry-level salaries, but also fairly graduated increases based on expanded roles in patient care, excellence in clinical practice, and leadership in directing the nursing staff to higher professional performance. In short, we must pay (and otherwise reward) nurses more to stay in practice than we pay them to abandon it—if we are ever to have a professional career in any meaningful sense of that term.

3 *There will be, in 1978, a congress or other interorganizational group of nursing associations that will plan and act collectively to present nursing's goals and functions to the public and to other health organizations.*

During the sixties, the National Commission became increasingly aware of the dynamic growth of specialty practice groups in professional nursing. There had been associations of operating room nurses, school nurses, and occupational health nurses for many years, but the rapid development of clinical nurse groups in critical care, obstetrics, emergency care, and a host of other fields represented a whole new force for involvement of nurses in the professional enhancement of their own practice and in the broader concerns and issues of the health care system.

Some traditionalists were disposed to dismiss these new associations as splinter groups that deflected their members from joining older, established organizations. Sheer force of numbers, however, argued that cooperation rather than indifference had to be the prevailing wisdom. In 1973, the American Association of Critical-Care Nurses issued an invitation to all the organizations whose membership was primarily composed of nurses to meet in San Clemente to discuss the formation of some type of congress or federation. The National Commission strongly endorsed this action and sent letters of support urging the organizations to send representatives to the meeting. Out of this beginning has emerged the federation of Nurse Specialty Organizations and the American Nurses' Association, which has assumed an interorganizational role.

From this federation has come much that is progressive and positive. The associations have exchanged information and viewpoints on certification, continuing education, and scope of practice. Cooperation has taken place between several of these groups and related elements within the ANA in developing joint approaches toward certification testing and recognition; unfortunately, some of these efforts have been suspended or terminated because basic disagreements could not always be resolved. Most important, however, is the fact that the foundation stones are in place for the future erection of a single House of Nursing that can bring diversity and common causes together.

In 1975, the former staff of the National Commission was able to obtain a commitment for a grant to establish an ad hoc planning committee to examine the objectives of the federation and to suggest a long-term plan for goals and activities. This offer was declined largely because the member organizations were still grappling with the early mechanics of cooperation and were very dubious of anything that smacked of a superorganization for nursing. Perhaps the time may now be better for the planning and establishment of some continuing procedure for working on the federation's goals and policies on a protracted basis.

Despite its limitations and its infrequent gatherings, the federation provides the beginning vehicle that the National Commission envisaged in 1970. There is now an interorganizational group that can present nursing's goals and functions more widely and effectively than ever before. With vision and collaboration, the federation can serve a vital function in the future.

4 *There will be, in 1978, a significant increase in the number of programs offering a combined L.P.N./R.N. program and a significant increase in the number of R.N. programs that offer special programs to meet the needs of L.P.N.s wishing to become R.N.s.*

In 1970, the National Commission urged special consideration of the aspirations of licensed practical or vocational nurses (V.N.s) to enroll in programs leading to the registered nurse license. It was the feeling of the Commission that the associate degree programs for nursing could effectively provide for the short-term solution of this need by offering advanced placement and special programming and, later, could present a long-term solution by developing a curricular pattern in which the first year of the associate degree program would provide an individual student with the tools for successfully passing the L.P.N. examination with the option of going directly on to the R.N. level through completion of the associate degree.

This study staff can now report that the educational aspects of upward mobility for licensed practical nurses seem to be essentially resolved. More than three-quarters of the associate degree programs responding to our survey indicated that they have planned programs for the admission and advanced placement of licensed practical nurses, and an increasing number of community colleges were adopting an articulated curriculum that permits any student to meet the essentials of an L.P.N. program in the first year of the A.D.N. program. Undoubtedly, there are localities and regions in which improvements in mobility are needed, but the general pattern is established and quite broadspread.

If there are continuing problems in articulation between licensed and registered nurses, they are likely to be political rather than educational. Several L.P./V.N. organizations encourage their members to retain their current status and have argued that L.P.N.s are the "real" bedside nurses whereas R.N.s are administrators and not practitioners. The kernel of truth that lies within traditional staffing expectations in hospitals and nursing homes does give some substance to these claims, but the emergent role expectations for registered nurses will challenge their validity. The situation is not ameliorated by the fact that salary levels for practical nursing have grown faster than those of registered nurses and that the financial incentive for pursuing upward mobility has been reduced by the realities of the marketplace.

5 *There will be, in 1978, a significant increase in the number of institutions offering programs designed for arts and sciences graduates, and there will be a significant increase in the variety of forms such programs will take.*

The first portion of this projection would appear to be substantially correct. Our survey of baccalaureate institutions for nursing education indicates that large numbers of arts and sciences graduates have applied for admission to degree programs in nursing—because of the recession, shrinking job opportunities in many fields of employment, and related occupational concerns. So general has this trend been that arts and sciences people are no longer exceptional in a nursing class, and many of the reporting colleges and universities feel that they have now established policies and procedures for facilitating the admission and placement of these particular students.

The second portion of the projection, however, has not been realized. Most arts and science graduates are admitted as advanced students in a second baccalaureate program. Although there are certainly academic precedents for this approach, the National Commission strongly urged the adoption of a master of arts degree in nursing as a preferable preparatory designation. The success of the experimental program at New York Medical College suggests that a graduate degree will be of additional drawing power to nontraditional applicants and more nearly represents parity with professional programs in education, health sciences, and behavioral sciences, which offer an alternative master's degree as an entry-level route to the profession.*

For several years, nursing has had increased experience with arts and sciences graduates from a variety of academic disciplines. Their strength, capacity, and motivation have been noted with enthusiasm by nursing faculty and educational administrators. This study staff would encourage greater experimentation with graduate preparatory programs to further the attractiveness of nursing, as well as combined-degree programs that might lead on to doctoral study and an increased capacity for research.

6   *There will be, in 1978, a significant number of states requiring as a condition for renewal of the nursing license, evidence of continued learning, maintenance of clinical skills, and/or related professional capacity.*

In 1973, there were no states that required evidence of clinical competence or of continuing education as an essential for renewal of the nursing license. Our survey of state nurses' associations in 1978 indicated that three states had mandated demonstration of clinical competence whereas nine states had instituted provisions for requiring continuing education credit. Many of these programs, however, have not been implemented because of the need to gear up educational programs, develop systems for recording the completion of learning units, and handle the myriad of administrative details that are required for maintenance of such a program.

Certainly, a beginning has been made toward the implementation of systematic reexamination of qualifications for license renewal. The experience of the first states to enact these requirements should be closely monitored to determine whether

*An interesting departure is the new doctoral program in nursing at Case-Western Reserve, which is intended for baccalaureate graduates of nonnursing programs. Thus the "first" nursing degree will be the doctorate.

statutory requirements are necessary or whether some combination of governmental, professional, and institutional approaches might not be preferable. The passage of a certification program monitored by a specialty practice organization or the ANA, for example, might be accepted as proof of continuing clinical competency. Likewise, completion of an advanced practitioner or clinical specialist program could be accepted upon endorsement by an institution for higher education. In recognizing the essential responsibility for the state to assure consumers of health care that a practitioner is safe and competent, it does not necessarily follow that a variety of cooperating agencies might not provide the best overall means for assessing that clinical competency.

The National Council of State Boards of Nursing should exercise a strong leadership role in the evaluation of current methods of relicensure and should examine ways in which this process can be made more effective and more efficient through both public and private participation. Particular attention should be directed at the significant increase in for-profit agencies whose sole activity seems to be the provision of continuing education programs for nurses. Adequate measures of quality and validity must be assured.

7 *There will be, in 1978, through professional and interprofessional planning, a systematic process for determining and certifying advanced levels of clinical skill among nurse practitioners.*

In 1970, the National Commission suggested that the American Academy of Nursing might be the agency to designate which bodies would take responsibility for certifying advanced levels of practice. Later, two changes on the organizational scene in nursing altered this proposal. The Academy of Nursing became essentially an honorary society for recognizing outstanding individuals who have contributed uniquely to the professional development of nursing. This function is significantly different from the clinical involvement originally proposed for the academy. At the same time, the emergence of the Federation of Specialty Nursing Organizations and the ANA brought into focus a wholly new apparatus for designating and endorsing groups to handle certification.

As of 1978, this study staff found remarkable progress in the development of certification procedures for advanced clinical levels in nursing. The Congress for Nursing Practice of the ANA through its Divisions on Practice has moved to establish testing and certification procedures. Similarly, several of the specialty practice groups are already in the process of certification, and more are intending to undertake the development of advanced recognition.

What has not occurred, however, is the expansion of cooperative approaches toward the designation of a single agency responsible for the certification of a given set of practitioners. The National Commission strongly urged the establishment of joint and multiple interdisciplinary bodies that would include the ANA and the relevant specialty practice group or groups; the Nurses' Association of the American College of Obstetricians and Gynecologists and the American College of Nurse Midwives, for example, have some overlapping clinical concerns, and both relate to the ANA Division on Maternal and Child Practice. Considerable difficulty, however, has been found in working out such cooperative arrangements, and, quite recently, at least two of the specialty practice groups have formally withdrawn from joint certification activities with the ANA. The issue is still of concern to all involved, and the ANA is currently studying how specialty practice certification might be recognized by the American Nurses' Association.

The possibility of jurisdictional disputes and competitive certification procedures is so proximate that this study staff strongly urges the Federation of Specialty Nursing Organizations and the ANA to assume responsibility for clarifying and systematizing procedures for certification and for designating agencies to assume responsibility and authority for carrying out professional recognition programs.* Organizational prerogatives and territory are insufficient excuses for not meeting the full professional responsibility the public has a right to expect from organized nursing. A concerted approach to certification of advanced practitioners is absolutely essential to the development of career perspectives and advanced role development in client care. Nursing must prove its ability to solve these internal problems with vision and firmness.

A SUMMARY STATEMENT

On balance, considerable progress has been made in most areas of the National Commission's recommendations for nursing roles, education, and careers. On the selected dimensions of 21 specific proposals, the evidence is that some have been realized in full, most have been accomplished in large part, and a small number have suffered from insufficient implementation.

It must be recognized that the entire thrust of the National Commission's *Abstract for Action* was designed to galvanize nursing into a strong and unambiguous profession capable of taking its place as a full principal in the partnerhood of health care organizations. Thus, the development of master planning and joint practice committees, the reformulation of educational curricula, and the reorganization of reward and recognition systems are all part and parcel of a design to ensure that nursing enters the twenty-first century prepared to meet its challenges without the impediments that have frustrated its development over the past 50 years.

The National Commission for the Study of Nursing and Nursing Education never presumed to say where nursing should be in the years ahead. What we attempted to do was to ensure that the known limitations of the past would be eliminated and a new professional pattern would be allowed to emerge unimpaired by the mistakes of an earlier society. The national concern for health as well as illness, the growing awareness of our blind spots toward women as professionals, and the increasing demonstration of maturity and clinical competence by individual nurses have led to a nationwide reappraisal of this profession. Increasingly we have

*It may well be that the proposed Nursing Credentialing Center might be the ultimate repository of such professional responsibility. Cooperative action, however, should not be put off until the NCC is established—if, indeed, it is.

begun to provide nursing with the armamentarium required to meet the needs that our society imposes.

This evaluative study and summary report documents the fact that considerable and significant progress has been made on the agenda proposed by the National Commission. It also documents that fact that there are still areas that must be addressed if nursing is truly going to keep its rendezvous with the twenty-first century. Among the most critical of the unfinished concerns are these:

1   In the area of nursing roles and functions, nursing with the help of others must continue the development of research and experimentation to enlarge its knowledge base and to improve its ability to enhance patient care.

2   In the area of education, total professional support must be directed to the establishment of a collegiate system for nursing education with concomitant enlargement of advanced clinical and research training.

3   In the area of careers, nursing must develop systematic procedures for recognizing and certifying advanced clinical competence and must press for new patterns of compensation that reward our best practitioners for staying in client care.

Taken all together, these proposals for the completion of the Commission agenda can be seen as the development of a corpus of scientific knowledge that can be transmitted through a systematic educational process to ensure a cadre of professional practitioners motivated and capable of delivering a variety and quality of client care that is beyond our abilities of today. If any one of these elements is neglected, American nursing will have failed in its opportunity and American society will be denied that quality of care that it has every right to expect. More than ever before, the choice is truly up to nursing. The tools have been made available, the plans arc drawn, but only nursing can crect this profcssional house which will end forever the ambiguity of its commitment and strength of will. The longer the delay on important issues, the weaker the resolve to act and the less the likelihood of full professionalism.

In 1970, the National Commission prepared an abstract of the directions to be taken toward the improvement of health care through the full utilization of nursing's potential. In that year, too, the Commission rejected the easy prospect of allowing its report to serve as the only guide to the future it had projected. For 3 years, ending in 1973, the Commission sought to put into motion the agencies, organizations, and guidelines that could encourage and assist the actual initiation of change and reformulation. This evaluation has attempted to measure the degree of implementation continued after the legal termination of the Commission as a focal point for action. The record is good; in some dimensions it is excellent. In critical respects, however, we are still short of our goals, still failing in our objectives for this our largest clinical health profession.

It is hoped that this report will serve as an encouragement and a stimulus. It should be an encouragement to all those in and out of nursing who helped to push this "locomotive" of a concept along the tracks to its destination. It should be a stimulus to that one more effort, that one more resolution, that one more accomplishment which can bring us to our appointed destiny. We are more than three-quarters of the way along the journey to full professionalism and partnerhood in the health care system; among the emergent leaders of nursing, many of whom were students when *An Abstract for Action* called for the fulfillment of their latent contributions to a wiser, better and more human pattern for client care, are the individuals who can realize the dream that was dreamt in so many hearts. May theirs be the everlasting satisfaction of that accomplishment.

REFERENCES

1 Jerome P. Lysaught (ed.), *Action in Nursing: Progress in Professional Purpose,* McGraw-Hill Book Company, New York, 1974, p. 135.
2 *Together: A Casebook of Joint Practices in Primary Care,* The National Joint Practice Commission, Chicago, 1977.
3 Virginia C. Hall, *Statutory Regulation of the Scope of Nursing Practice—A Critical Survey,* The National Joint Practice Commission, 1975.
4 *NJPC Bulletin,* vol. 4, no. 2, December 1978, p. 9.
5 Ibid., pp. 17–18.
6 Laurian M. Whyte, "The Effect of Certification on the Wages and Hours Worked by Critical Care Nurses," unpublished doctoral thesis, The University of Rochester, Rochester, N.Y., 1979, pp. 67ff.
7 *Report of the American Hospital Association's Advisory Panel on Nurse Shortage,* American Hospital Association, Chicago, June 6, 1979.
8 *NJPC Bulletin,* op. cit., pp. 11–12.
9 Jerome P. Lysaught, *You Can Get There from Here: The Orange County/Long Beach Experiment in Improved Patterns of Nursing Education,* The University of Rochester, Rochester, N.Y., 1979.
10 Patricia T. Haase, *A Proposed System for Nursing: Theoretical Framework,* part 2, Southern Regional Education Board, Atlanta, 1976.
11 Whyte, op. cit.